'Demographic change is the most neglected shaper of our future. Camilla Cavendish has written the most interesting, perceptive and iconoclastic guide to its many implications. This is a truly important book.'

LAWRENCE SUMMERS, President Emeritus and
Charles W. Eliot University Professor of Harvard University

'As deeply inspirational as it is informative. If you want to know how to live a long, vibrant life, *Extra Time* is a must-read.'

DR DAVID SINCLAIR, Geneticist, Author of *Lifespan*

'A great book: it summarises the key principles that every government and society needs to adopt to help people live longer better, with less dementia and frailty.'

SIR MUIR GRAY, former Chief Knowledge Officer
to the National Health Service

'*Extra Time* offers a clear-eyed view of the challenges and opportunities of longer lives and rapidly shifting age demography. As we enter what the World Health Organization defines as the "Decade of Healthy Ageing", Camilla Cavendish makes a compelling, urgent, and highly readable case for change.'

PAUL IRVING, Chairman, Milken Institute
Center for the Future of Aging

'*Extra Time* should perhaps be called "About Time" because it is a long overdue and brilliant counterpoint to all those pervasive arguments that our ageing societies will be poorer and sadder. Growing old, as individuals and nations, need not mean growing frailer and duller. Camilla Cavendish has written an empowering and important manifesto for how an older society can be a better society.' ROBERT PESTON

'In this remarkable and frequently optimistic book Camilla Cavendish sets out what is part warning and part redefinition of what it is to live longer. Her statistics and her observations of how differently rich and poor will age are breathtaking. But it is above all her bravery in challenging our very notions of ageing that makes this a must-read book for all those struggling to understand the enormity of change that longer life now brings.' EMILY MAITLIS

'*Extra Time* by Camilla Cavendish is an optimistic, uplifting and practical book about the huge potential for humans to live not just longer lives, but more fulfilling lives. An inspiring and essential read.' ARIANNA HUFFINGTON

'You will want to read this book: it is about how we could all grow older and stay fitter. Camilla Cavendish has trawled labs across America, Japan and Europe to discover the latest developments in the many ways of ageing … she sets out her findings with clarity and enthusiasm. More than this, she addresses the social and political dimensions of how best to share these benefits among us all. A welcome and optimistic voice.' JOAN BAKEWELL

'[Camilla's] approach is a societal one, making convincing arguments for public health changes as well as suggesting ways we can improve our own chances.' *Daily Express*

'A well-informed policy manual on how an older society can be a better society.' *Evening Standard*

EXTRA TIME

10 LESSONS
for
LIVING LONGER BETTER

Camilla Cavendish

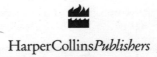

HarperCollins*Publishers*

HarperCollins*Publishers*
1 London Bridge Street
London SE1 9GF

www.harpercollins.co.uk

First published by HarperCollins*Publishers* 2019
This edition published 2020

3 5 7 9 10 8 6 4 2

Text © Camilla Cavendish 2019
Illustrations © HarperCollins*Publishers* 2019

Camilla Cavendish asserts the moral right to be
identified as the author of this work

A catalogue record of this book is
available from the British Library

ISBN 978-0-00-829517-2

Printed and bound in Great Britain by
CPI Group (UK) Ltd, Croydon

MIX
Paper from
responsible sources
FSC™ C007454

This book is produced from independently certified FSC™ paper
to ensure responsible forest management.

For more information visit: www.harpercollins.co.uk/green

In memory of Richard Cavendish,
1930–2016

Contents

Introduction

The New World of Extra Time

IN 2018, A DUTCHMAN began a court battle to make himself legally 20 years younger. Emile Ratelband, 69, told a court in Arnhem in the Netherlands that he did not feel 'comfortable' with his official chronological age, which did not reflect his emotional state – and was preventing him from finding work, or love online. He wanted to change his date of birth from 11 March 1949 to 11 March 1969.

Doctors had told him that his body was that of a 45-year-old, Ratelband argued. 'When I'm 69,' he said, 'I am limited. If I'm 49, I can take up more work. When I'm on Tinder and it says I'm 69, I'm outdated.' His friends had urged him to lie, he claimed, but 'if you lie, you have to remember everything you say'.

Ratelband compared his quest to be identified as younger with that of people who wish to be identified as transgender – implying that age should be fluid. He said his parents were dead, so could not be upset by his desire to turn back the clock. He even offered to waive his right to a pension.

Ratelband, a 'positivity coach', is a provocateur who enjoys attention. The court turned him down, ruling that an age change would have 'undesirable implications' for legal rights, such as the right to vote. But this seemingly frivolous case actually illustrates something profound: we are on the cusp of an entirely new period in our history, which is coming at us fast.

This is the advent of Extra Time.

If you are in your fifties or sixties today, you have a very good chance of living into your nineties. If you play your cards right and have luck on your side, many of those years could be healthy and productive. Our chronological age is becoming decoupled from our biological capabilities.

In football, 'extra time' is the period when *there's everything still to play for.* That will be true for many of us. Droves of people are 'unretiring' and going back to work. Advances in biology and neuroscience will help us stay younger longer. But our institutions, and our societies, have not caught up. Ratelband's looks, his physical strength, his ambitions are out of kilter with what we traditionally associate with being 69. He feels compelled to go to the extreme lengths of changing his birth date. Why can't we, instead, just change our view of what it means to be 69?

The Fierce Urgency of 100

In 1917, King George V of England sent the first ever telegram to a centenarian. It was handwritten, and delivered by bicycle. In 2017, Queen Elizabeth II sent out thousands of 100th birthday cards, with a team of seven employed to administer them all.[1]

The era of Extra Time will see a growing number of centenarians. The Office for National Statistics estimates that one in three babies born in Britain today will live to 100. Some scientists even think we could live to 150 (as we will see in Chapter 6).

This should be a fairy tale. Instead, there are widespread fears that we are sitting on a 'demographic time bomb', with droves of elderly people about to bankrupt governments and hurt GDP. If people get less creative as they age, and stop work around 60, economies could slump and younger generations could face crippling taxes.

But it doesn't have to be that way. More and more people, like Emile Ratelband, have no desire to retire. Fears about the declining ratio of workers to pensioners rest on the official definition of 'working age', as 15–64. But David Hockney became the world's foremost iPad painter at 76; Tina Turner made the cover of *Vogue* at 73; Yuichiro Miura climbed Everest aged 80. Warren Buffett is still investing in his eighties and David Attenborough is making hit TV series in his nineties. Behind them stride loads of ordinary people who see Extra Time as an opportunity, who are starting businesses and are highly productive. They can defuse the time bomb.

Will they be fit enough? When a football match goes into Extra Time, there's a premium on fitness. Here, the omens are pretty good. Today's seventy-somethings are sprightlier than ever before, and the incidence of dementia is falling. There is work to do, though, on health inequalities. Increases in life expectancy have slowed in the UK,[2] where the average life expectancy at birth is now 82 for women and nudging 80 for men. In America, life expectancy at birth has dropped for three years in a row,[3] partly because of the opioid epidemic. Both countries face a battle against obesity – and poverty (see pages 19 and 23).[4]

Globally, demographers think these dips in life expectancy are probably blips. The twenty-first century will be defined by people living longer, in societies which are growing older much faster than we have fully realised. But are they ageing faster? Only if you cling to out-of-date notions of what it means to be 50, 65 or 80.

Islands of Extra Time

On the Pacific island of Okinawa, there is no word for retirement. The longest-living women in the world are still caring for great-grandchildren when they hit their 100s. Okinawans are rarely lonely, because they are supported by a network of friends, the '*moai*', who are committed to share both good times and bad. The typical Okinawan house doesn't have much furniture: people tend to eat sitting on the floor, so they are getting up and down many times a day. They also have a strong sense of '*ikigai*', roughly translated as 'reason for being'. My Japanese friends tell me that you find your *ikigai* at the place where your values intersect with what you enjoy doing, and what you are good at.

Okinawa is one of the Blue Zones, the parts of the world identified by researcher Dan Buettner, where people have low rates of chronic disease and live exceptionally long lives. While it's not possible to distil a single magic ingredient, common to all Blue Zones are plant-based diets with very little processed food, strong friendships and a sense of purpose, lots of sleep and strenuous physical activity.

We can't all live on islands, getting up with the sun and tilling the soil. But the Blue Zones do suggest that what we think of as 'normal' may be a very poor version of what our natural selves could be. And that is incredibly positive.

Why I Wrote This Book

I started writing this book in 2016, after my beloved father died. He had dreaded getting 'old', so much so that it whittled down his life much too early. I remember his gloom on his fiftieth birthday. As we sat together on his favourite cliff in Cornwall, watching the waves break below, he said he felt that everything was 'over'. I was a child, and 50 was older than I could imagine. But I did notice, from that point on, that my father started to think of himself in a different way. He would say 'Oh, I'm too old for that' with a sigh. After my mother left him, he refused to get a cat, although he adored them, on the basis that it might outlive him and be left homeless. He was 58 when he got divorced, and missed our two cats, Arthur and Merlin, most terribly (they went with my mother in the divorce, along with a hotly contested dining table). He ended up living, in largely excellent health, to 86. And he lived all that time without cats, who could have kept him company.

After he died, I couldn't stop thinking about the way age can become a barrier.

My mother lied about her age until she was 72, because she was terrified she would lose her job as a secretary, and default on the mortgage she took out after the divorce. This created a huge burden of deception. She never dared join the company pension scheme for fear of being found out. She also hated the feeling that, as her looks dwindled, she was becoming invisible. She refused to let my children call her 'Granny', or refer to her in any way as a grandmother, which made things awkward between them.

In conventional terms, my parents were 'old' – almost 40 – by the time they conceived me. They'd met at Oxford University in the 1950s, she a glamorous American who'd grown up in Greenwich, Connecticut, he the bookish son of an English vicar. Their world was an intellectual, bohemian one of artists and academics for whom work was passion, savings in the bank negligible and 'retirement' anathema. My father dictated his final article for *History Today* magazine from a bed in Charing Cross Hospital. My mother was campaigning to help a friend get his job back when she had her final heart attack.

My thoughts about my parents chimed with my growing professional awareness of our fatalism about older people. As a journalist, and through my work for the Department of Health, I have met many compassionate nursing and care staff struggling against tick-box cultures and low pay.[5] When I sat on the board of our national hospital and care-home regulator,[6] it was clear that patients were being warehoused in post-war silos. As head of the Number 10 Policy Unit, I worked to introduce the sugar tax and other measures to combat obesity, a condition which is making people old before their time, but is portrayed as a 'choice'. And I felt that media excitement about living to 100 jarred with a lack of ambition about what that should mean.

I have written this book to challenge our notions of ageing, and find out what different countries are doing to build a new world for Extra Time. I have been privileged to meet many wonderful pioneers, who I think of as 'rebels against fate', who are refusing to dress demurely, stop work or be carted off to care homes.

The rebels against fate intuitively understand that something fundamental has changed. They are all saying, in different ways, that age should not define us. My goal in this book is to spread their message, to persuade you to contemplate your own future before it's too late, and to try to change the pattern of thinking in our societies about what we mean by 'old'. Because it sure as hell isn't 50, whatever my father thought. Yet much of the data about the 'old' still starts at 50 – when some of us will be only halfway through our lives.

This book is not a rose-tinted rhapsody. I don't predict that we will all be skipping our way cheerfully to 120. In fact, I've written it partly as a warning.

Living longer is not a blessing, in my view, unless it is living better for longer. Neither of my parents had any desire to live to 100. What they cared about was living as full a life as possible, and then hopefully checking out as fast as possible.

One of the most shocking things I have confirmed, in researching this book, is just how drastically the futures of the rich and poor, the highly educated and the less educated are diverging. Only Japan has begun to effectively address the health problems which mean that some people are what the Japanese call 'Young-Old' at 80, while others are 'Old-Old' at 65. For me, this is one of the biggest ethical challenges of our time. If we don't fix it, the rich, the educated and the lucky may still be thriving at 90 – but they will be living in societies which cannot afford to look after those who are less fortunate. We must prevent that from happening: since one measure of a civilised society is how it treats its elderly.

A Different, Better World

This book spans many aspects of a huge topic. I have tried to break it down into ten lessons, each of which reflects what I have learned from experts, academics and policymakers, but also from those on the frontline. I've interviewed biologists who are challenging the very notion that ageing is inevitable; neuroscientists who are finding ways to stave off brain decline; and social entrepreneurs who are working to bring the generations together, rather than letting them drift apart.

I begin by surveying the demographic trends, longer lives and plummeting birth rates, which pose a profound and unexpected challenge to our species. Voluntary childlessness was always presumed to be evolutionarily impossible. But birth rates are falling so fast that some countries will soon shrink. China is growing old before it gets rich. If America stays vibrant, this could alter the geopolitical balance of power.

Almost without noticing, we have created an entirely new stage of life – an extended middle age. I look at this new stage in Chapter 2, and at how the media, and governments, send the wrong signals. I look at alternative ways to compute healthy lifespan, and at the widening gap between the rich and educated, and the less fortunate. In Chapter 3 I explore what true biological ageing might look like, without junk food and sedentary lifestyles, and argue that obesity is making some people old before their time. I am not advocating any particular product or medicine in this book, but I do suggest that the evidence for aerobic exercise, and against sugar, is compelling.

Some Silicon Valley billionaires are on a quest to find immortality. Their research is fascinating. Especially intriguing are the 'super-centenarians', whose risk of dying levels off after the age of 105. But my chief interest is in improving life, not prolonging it. In Chapter 5 I describe developments in neuroscience which show that we are never too old to learn. I look at what kinds of brain training might help keep us sharp, and at the 'cognitive reserve' which may be protective against Alzheimer's. In Chapter 6 I hunt down pills which claim to have anti-ageing properties, harnessing genes and proteins in our bodies. These discoveries raise what may sound like an odd question: should we treat ageing as a disease? But in another decade it may seem eccentric to treat one illness at a time, rather than to use the underlying circuits in our bodies to ward off many different conditions.

That doesn't mean we won't get ill. In Chapter 8 I meet cold but useful robots in Japan, and warm inspiring nurses in Holland, and I argue for more compassionate health and care systems based on a blend of technology and humanity.

The challenge for CEOs is considerable. The multi-generational workforce is on the way, but it will not be straightforward to manage. Even though jobs are being automated, retiring babyboomers are creating skill shortages. We need a fourth stage of education, to match the fourth industrial revolution. Luckily, pioneers are shrugging off the notion that retirement is good for you, and are starting successful businesses (Chapter 4). Others are creating the kinds of neighbourhoods we will all need, to look after each other (Chapter 7). Still others are harnessing the energy and altruism of older people to do good, whether that is grandmothers in Zimbabwe or hospital volunteers in England (Chapter 9).

Longer lives, and shrinking numbers of young people, are putting pressure on the social contract. How will our societies look after the old, without bankrupting the young? In Chapter 8 I propose a new settlement for funding social care, drawing on the examples of Germany and Japan. In Chapter 10 I argue that the new divide is not simply between young and old, but between the skilled and the less skilled, at all ages.

One of the greatest blocks to progress is our own prejudice. We need to transform our attitudes, and realise it's not old age that's getting longer, it's middle age. The challenge is urgent. The world is becoming an older one, faster than anyone anticipated. That's not only because we are living longer, it's also because of what I call the 'Death of Birth', as described in the next chapter.

1

The Death of Birth

Demography tips the balance of power

BY 2020, FOR THE first time in history, there will be more people on the planet over 65 than under 5.[1] More grandparents than grandchildren.

Two trends are driving this ageing of the world. First, we are living longer. In the twentieth century, average life expectancy increased by 30 years in most developed countries, because of better nutrition and sanitation, and medical advances. Men currently live longest in Switzerland, with an average life expectancy at birth of 82; women live longest in Japan, to about 87. Australia, Israel, Canada, South Korea and most Western European countries are close behind. The gap between men and women is narrowing, because men who once led rackety lives (drinking and smoking) are cleaning up their act.

The second reason is that the world's women are turning away from motherhood. In 1964 the average woman had just over 5 children; in 2015 she had only 2.5.[2]

There are now 83 countries, home to nearly half the world's population, with fertility rates below the 'replacement rate' – roughly 2.1 births per woman – needed to maintain the population. Australia, New Zealand, Brazil, Chile and almost every country in Europe now has fertility below that level. South Africa and India are moving rapidly towards replacement rate, with birth rates of 2.5 and 2.3 respectively.[3]

The changes will alter the shape of countries. Japan's population is already shrinking. By the middle of this century Italy, Poland, South Korea and Russia will be dwindling too.[4] And these shifts could redraw the geopolitical balance of power: between countries on an ageing, shrinking trajectory – notably China – and countries which are sustained by younger, immigrant populations – currently the US.

Africa will provide the young of the future. The populations of 26 African countries are expected to double between 2017 and 2050, adding another 1.3 billion people to that continent.[5]

Fewer humans should be good news for the environment, once global population peaks (some time after 2070, though estimates range from 9 to 11 billion).[6] But the impact on humans can already be glimpsed. Visit Japan's Akita Prefecture, where over a third of residents are over 65 and the main growth industry is funeral parlours.[7] Or go to Rudong in eastern China, where half the schools have closed in the past 15 years as the younger generation moves away.

Demography is changing not only the landscape, but the very meaning of family. What networks will we rely on, as children become scarce?

The Chinese government has passed an 'Elderly Rights Law', threatening to fine children who don't visit parents often enough.[8] But the children are fighting back. 'What is considered "often"?' complained one poster on Weibo, the Chinese Twitter.[9] 'It's fine that no one is paying for us to visit our parents, but is there someone who can give us time off to do it?' asked another, refusing to buy into traditional notions of family.

The best way to visualise what is happening is through the population pyramids used by demographers. In 1950, if you laid out the population of any nation with each age group represented by a bar, the youngest at the bottom and the oldest at the top, it looked like a pyramid, with the young outnumbering the old. That has been the shape throughout recorded history, as this chart for Japan shows:

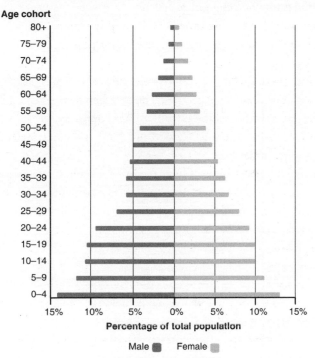

Population of Japan by age and sex in 1950

Age cohort

Percentage of total population

Male ■ Female ▨

Since then, falling birth rates and longer lifespans have changed the picture dramatically. Japan, the world's oldest society, has one of the lowest birth rates in the world: 1.4 births per woman. Fifty years ago, life expectancy in Japan was about 72 years. Now it is 84. In 2015, over a quarter of the population was over 65, turning the pyramid into a barrel:

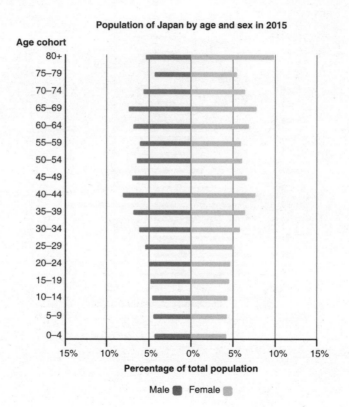

Population of Japan by age and sex in 2015

Between now and 2050, longer lifespans will continue to alter the pyramids' shape. The fastest growing group in the world population will be those aged over 80. In Japan, the pyramid will stretch up and outwards, to look more like a flowerpot:

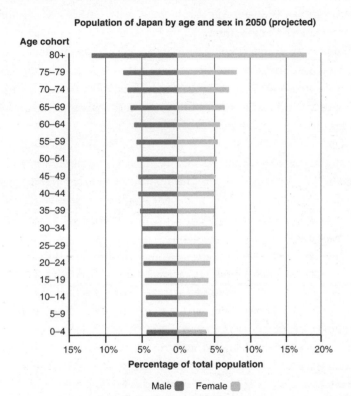

Population of Japan by age and sex in 2050 (projected)

One former health minister has predicted that 'the Japanese race will become extinct'. The first question is why? Why have millions of individuals simultaneously changed their minds about having children?

Japan: 'Herbivore Men' and Career Women

'Men here don't want a woman who's cleverer than them,' says Keiko, a Japanese executive in her early forties, who is wearing a smart suit and demure heels when we meet in the lobby of the Tokyo Hilton. 'They worry you might be demanding, that you might be demanding in bed too. And I just think, why bother? Why bother with a guy who's more interested in his Xbox?'

Something strange is going on in Japan, which now has the world's highest proportion of old people. In 2013, it was claimed, more nappies were sold for elderly, incontinent people than for babies.[10] That ugly benchmark proclaims the raw truth: babies have gone out of fashion.

The roots of this shift, in a society which has traditionally prized family above everything, lie in a feminist revolution: women are shaking off the traditions of dutiful service to husband and household, and challenging men to adapt. 'I wouldn't mind a child, if I'm honest,' said a Japanese student I met in London. 'But I'm not sure I'd want to put up with a husband.'

'It's hard,' says one Japanese woman in her late thirties, who speaks perfect English and has married a New Zealander. 'Many of my friends are really serious about their careers. It's their chance and they're not going to bother with a man who can't bring home the bacon.'

As women become more ambitious for themselves, they talk disparagingly about what they call 'herbivore men' (so¯shoku-kei danshi), a term coined in 2006 by the Nikkei columnist Maki Fukasawa. The herbivore man doesn't know how to ask a woman out on a date. He's intimidated by women. And, the implication is, he's not even that interested. A survey in the *Japan Times* found 20 per cent of men in their late twenties reported having little or no interest in sex – some citing crippling long working hours.[11]

It's not clear to what extent the stereotype is true. There are still plenty of Love Hotels, the Japanese hotels which were created for salarymen to grab some respite. And the number of children produced by married couples is still hovering around replacement rate. But far more people are staying single. As arranged marriages disappear, hundreds of thousands of men whose mothers would once have found them a bride are struggling to adapt. One in four 50-year-old Japanese men has never been married.[12] Since this is a country which still feels uncomfortable having children out of wedlock, that's bad for birth.

Having children is also a costly business. In surveys, 20- and thirty-something men and women[13] say lack of money is a serious obstacle to getting married. Couples increasingly need two incomes. But it's hard to combine a career with motherhood in a culture where people stay at their desks late.

Cost is not the whole story. Many women have been liberated from the need to find a husband to support them, as employers have become more open-minded about hiring. This partly stems, ironically, from the realisation that Japan must utilise all its talents if its economy is to prosper as the population shrinks. As all the curves on the graph turn downwards, experts are now looking desperately for solutions.

'We must increase immigration, or we will see our nation vanish,' says Dr Jun Saito, a leading economist at the UCLA Japan Center in Tokyo. Dr Saito believes that Japan must import more foreign workers even if it manages to increase the number of women and older people in the work force. 'Even if we raised the fertility rate to 2.1 tomorrow,' he tells me, 'an option that is difficult to achieve, the population would not stabilize until 60 to 70 years later.'

Japanese reluctance to admit immigrants is legendary. Fewer than 2 per cent of the country's workforce is foreign. Although the government recently created new visas for low-skilled foreign workers in industries like construction and care, and has broken a taboo by letting those workers bring their families immediately, rather than after five years, the numbers are a trickle. Only 18 foreign workers have qualified for the care-worker visa, partly because the exams are in Japanese.

'The worst scenario in my mind,' Dr Saito confides, 'is that even if we open up the country, nobody comes.'

China: Growing Old Before It Gets Rich

They call it the grey wall of China. By 2100, China's elderly population will dwarf that of any other country except India. It'll be so large, wags joke, that you'll be able to see it from outer space. At the park around Beijing's Temple of Heaven, in the cool of early morning, hundreds of older people are playing cards, doing tai-chi or exercising. A group of about 50, mainly women, dance to lilting music. They move gracefully, quietly, in a choreographed routine, on the paths between the trees.

It's an uplifting, harmonious scene. The women place their feet confidently, and with precision. But it's hard to feel so confident of the future. Most of the people in this park are retired. China's working-age population has been in decline since 2012[14] and is set to fall by almost a quarter by 2050. The demographer Nicholas Eberstadt, of the American Enterprise Institute, has predicted that this will drag down China's GDP growth rate. By mid-century, China's population could look much more like Japan's – but without Japan's affluence.

The birth rate was falling even before the government introduced the One-Child Policy in 1978. Now, China is awash with only children. Many find themselves having to support two parents and four grandparents – known as 'the 4-2-1' problem. There is the added, disturbing glut of bachelors because so many families preferred sons to daughters. These 'guang gun' (bare branches) will struggle to find brides.

Sensing the danger, the Communist Party dropped the One-Child Policy in 2015. But it is probably too late. Few eligible families have applied to have a second child. Many don't feel they can afford it, because so many have moved to cities where the cost of living is high.

Seven in ten Chinese mothers work, with little time for an extra child.

Marriage is becoming less attractive. On TV dating shows like *If You Are the One*, successful Chinese women criticise potential suitors for being ugly or poor. More women than men now attend Chinese universities, and many are defying the jibes about unmarried women being '*shengnu*', or 'leftover'. A survey by the Chinese dating website Baihe.com has found 75 per cent of women saying that any husband should earn twice as much as them.

The Chinese Academy of Social Sciences predicts that the Chinese population will peak at 1.44 billion in 2029 before entering 'unstoppable' decline.[15] By 2065, it says, the population will have shrunk to the levels of the mid-1990s.

What could this mean for China as a military power? Mark L. Haas, a political scientist at Duquesne University, Pittsburgh, Pennsylvania, has suggested that China could be forced to make 'geriatric peace' with other nations, as it becomes too burdened by its elderly to maintain military spending. That is not certain: China may not feel beholden to spend as much as a democracy on older citizens, and it can use technology to raise productivity. But it is too big to be able to level the playing field by importing enough immigrants.

Instead, the government has started offering five-year multiple-entry visas to tempt its diaspora back home – something South Africa and India are also doing.[16] It is also contemplating raising the retirement age, which is 60 for men and 55 for women.[17]

Will they be fit enough? China faces an increasing burden of chronic disease approaching Western levels. Junk food and stress have accompanied rapid urbanisation and the country has not yet broken the smoking habit. Under Mao, China's population was surprisingly healthy: it saw the world's most sustained increase in life expectancy, from 35 in 1949 to 65 in 1980.[18] That healthy, working-age population helped to drive its unprecedented economic growth.[19] But now, China is growing old with neither Japan's wealth nor its health, at a time when many of its jobs still require physical, manual labour. And its rival, America, is on a different path.

China v America

America has long been a demographic exception, with a higher birth rate than most other rich countries. China's population is currently around four times the size of America's. But that gap will have halved[20] by the end of this century, unless America slams the door shut on immigrants.

The chart below gives a glimpse into the geopolitics of the next few decades. It shows China's working-age population dropping, along with Europe's, while America's remains stable:

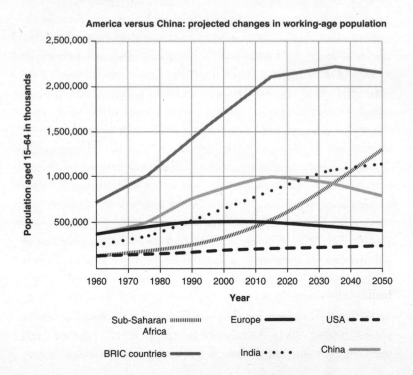

America versus China: projected changes in working-age population

Before the financial crisis, the American population was sustaining itself, with a birth rate of 2.12.[21] This is partly because it has higher levels of immigration, and because immigrants tend to have larger families. In the US, 23 per cent of births are to foreign-born women,[22] while only 13 per cent of the population is comprised of immigrants.[23]

American women also become mothers earlier than in any other OECD country: at an average age of 26, compared with 28 in the UK, and 31 in Italy. Only 14 per cent of US women remain childless, compared to 18 per cent in the UK and 23 per cent in Germany.[24]

There is a dark side. America has been lagging behind other rich countries in life expectancy, partly because its high rates of obesity mean it has failed to combat deaths from stroke. But now, US life expectancy at birth has dropped for three years in a row, the first drop since the AIDS/HIV epidemic, partly because of what the Princeton professors Case and Deaton have dubbed 'deaths of despair'[25] – from suicide, alcohol and opioids.[26] Poverty and inequality pose real challenges.

In 2017, America also hit a 40-year low in its fertility rate, of 1.76.[27] What is not clear is whether this is a post-crisis blip or a new direction. The fertility rate of Mexicans in America dropped by a third between 2006 and 2013, partly because of the financial squeeze – and it hasn't yet recovered. If migrants are to keep working their magic on fertility, they need to keep coming, because second- and third-generation immigrants tend to adopt the cultures of the host country and have fewer babies. Any president who builds a wall could therefore get more than he bargained for: because population is shaping up to be a powerful geopolitical weapon.

India: Educating Rhia

Today's Indian couples say their ideal family size is two children, according to a poll by *The Economist*.[28] That's smaller than the ideal family cited by Brits and Americans. Fifty years since the biologist Paul

Erhlich predicted mass famine in his book *The Population Bomb*, India's youthful population is growing slowly. The average woman now has just 2.3 children – fewer if she is Sikh, Jain or Christian, slightly more if she is Hindu and a bit more again if she is Muslim.

India did not need a One-Child Policy to reach this point. Although government has nudged people to have smaller families in various ways, India is a good advert for the principle that educating girls reduces the number of children they have. Especially if you accept that education comes in many forms. Birth rates have fallen where cable TV has arrived in rural areas, bringing Bollywood soap operas featuring independent childless women and chic urban mothers with small families.[29] Audiences name their babies after the characters, become less tolerant of domestic violence and use contraception. India is not alone: telenovelas have had a similar effect in Brazil.[30]

While India still wrestles with poverty and illiteracy, it seems that urbanisation, growing prosperity, public health and most of all education are powerful contraceptives.

Singapore: City Living

'Having kids was important to our parents,' one thirty-something civil servant in Singapore explained to researcher Joel Kotkin, who conducted extensive interviews with young professionals. 'But now we tend to have a cost and benefit analysis about family. The cost is tangible, but the benefits are not.'[31]

Such chilling pragmatism resonates in many parts of Asia, especially those where property prices are high. It is no accident that Singapore, Tokyo, Hong Kong, Shanghai and Beijing, some of the world's most expensive cities, have some of the lowest birth rates. The Singapore government's 'Marriage and Parenthood Package' offers substantial bonuses to couples who have children. But it's not working too well. Many ambitious youngsters seem more focused on their careers: a third of graduates aged 30 to 34 years old are single in Singapore, and the birth rate is 1.2.[32]

These modern workers don't seem to worry that no one will look after them in old age. Across Asia, the traditional model of close-knit families is breaking down. Social networks are increasingly made up of friends, not relatives: reinforcing the notion that childlessness is normal.

Europe: Waiting for Mr Right?

'Capitalism + atheism + feminism = sterility = migration,' tweeted Julian Assange, founder of WikiLeaks and fugitive from justice, in 2017. 'EU birthrate = 1.6,' he went on. 'Replacement = 2.1. Merkel, May, Macron, Gentiloni [the leaders of Germany, Britain, France and Italy at the time] all childless.'

This was a neat summary of Europe's plight. And nowhere does it apply more strongly than in Italy, which most of us still associate with large Catholic families. The country of '*amore*' now has the lowest birth rate in Europe. This is partly a consequence of youth unemployment. The long, grim recession since the financial crash of 2008 has seen many Italians travel abroad to find jobs, and others fearing they can't afford children.

The average Italian woman would still like two or more children.[33] But she doesn't have her first child until 31 – older than anywhere else in the EU.[34] One reason may be that two-thirds of Italian men under 35 are still living with their parents, in contrast to most young women.[35] Politicians have dubbed these Mama's boys '*bamboccioni*' ('big babies') who won't grow up. Political commentator Antonio Politi has claimed that women are being deterred from raising families by men who are neither fulfilling their roles as breadwinners, nor stepping up to fatherhood.

Attempts to warn women not to leave it too late have backfired spectacularly. When Italy's health minister Beatrice Lorenzin organised a national Fertility Day, with talks up and down the country, she was met with outraged counter-demonstrations. Women marched through the streets carrying placards reading '*siamo in attesa*':[36] a play on the Italian for 'we're expecting', which also translates as 'we're waiting'. Waiting for jobs, waiting for affordable childcare, and waiting for equality. Many Italian women still lose their jobs when they get pregnant; one in four is sacked within a year of having her first child.[37] Romance is not entirely dead, but the birth rate is in trouble when women need to work but don't have equality.

Germany has similarly high rates of childlessness to Italy. But in Europe's prosperous heart, this has less to do with money worries. 'In the days of "*Kinder, Küche, Kirche*" ["Children, Kitchen, Church"] it was natural to have children,' I'm told by Dr Jan Kessler, a paediatrician in Munich. 'But that's old-fashioned to a generation which wants to keep its options open. They want to study; they want a good career; it's never really a good time to have a child.'

Women are enjoying success, and don't always want to deal with old-fashioned views of motherhood. 'No one minds me having a career,' one married academic told me. 'But I would get a lot of flak if I left a child in a crèche.' Some German women fear being labelled as *Rabenmütter*, 'raven mothers', if they dare to combine work and motherhood. This appalling image, of ravens as carrion-eaters who neglect their young, seems to weigh heavily on some women, who are in any case not certain whether they want children.

The German government gives generous parental leave and has massively expanded day care. It now spends almost three times as much on benefits to families as it spends on defence.[38] (The UK spends about 1.3 times more.[39]) The reforms were led by Ursula von der Leyen, a government minister and mother of seven, who subsidised paternity leave and declared that men should be responsible for half of the childcare. And the birth rate has nudged up a little, with the help of immigrants. To keep pace, the Federal Statistical Office has estimated that the country would need half a million immigrants every year until 2040. That seems unlikely, given the backlash which followed Angela Merkel's opening the borders to around a million refugees in 2015.

The birth rate is higher in Britain, where part-time working and maternity benefits are routine. That's partly because of high levels of immigration: 28 per cent of live births in the UK are to foreign-born women,[40] though foreign-born people make up about 14 per cent of the population.

We are also breeding a nation of only children. Almost half of British families now contain only one child. It's not clear how much of that is deliberate. In polls, Brits say their ideal family is just over two children, but the birth rate is 1.76.

Sarah Davies, a teacher, was in her mid-thirties when she plucked up the courage to ask her long-term boyfriend to settle down. He dumped her. Now, she wonders if she's left it too late. 'No one will fancy me if I look desperate,' she says gloomily, staring at a dating site. Ms Davies is not one of those mythical creatures regularly accused by the UK press of ignorantly frittering away their fertility. She's been muffling the ticking of her biological clock for years, fearing men are on a different timetable. 'They've got no incentive,' she reflects. 'If I was a man, I'd probably focus on my career too, and not want to be hamstrung by a baby till I'd made it.' A lack of suitable partners may explain recent increases in the numbers of single women seeking IVF, and why birth rates for women over 40 are at their highest level since 1949.[41] That seems more likely than the idea that highly capable career women, who stick to every other timetable, somehow 'forgot' to have kids.

Is Life Expectancy Stalling?

Galloping increases in life expectancy have recently slowed dramatically in the UK, and to a lesser extent in Germany, Sweden and the Netherlands. This has surprised actuaries. Some blame it on government cuts to public services, although those were not uniform in those countries.[42] Others believe it has more to do with a slowdown in the incredible progress we have made against heart attacks and stroke.

Life expectancy at birth grew substantially during the twentieth century, because we were reducing deaths among infants and children: but life expectancy from the age of 65 barely budged. Between 1970 and 2011, however, older people saw a dramatic change: life expectancy at 65 increased 20 times as fast as in the previous century. The main reason? A massive drop in deaths from heart attack and stroke, driven by people giving up cigarettes.

Since 2011, progress has slowed. 'It's possible we have gone back to the time before 2000, when life expectancy improvement was more gradual,' says Gordon Aitken, insurance analyst at RBC Capital Markets. 'From 2000 to 2010, we saw the wealthier getting healthier. But it's hard to keep reducing deaths from cardiovascular diseases at the same rate. And obesity and diabetes are on the rise.'

There is no consensus on how the change affects different socio-economic groups. One data set suggests that the 'Comfortable' are unaffected, and that the losses are among the 'Hard-Pressed'. Another suggests that all groups are seeing a slowdown in improvement.[43]

While these differences are of enormous importance to insurers, because they affect annuity payouts, they are less crucial for the rest of us. Mr Aitken explains that the chance of dying in 2018, for example, didn't increase from the previous year. What has happened is that the forecasts for growth were too optimistic. A 65-year-old man in the UK is now expected to live to 86.5, while a 65-year-old woman is expected to reach 88.4.

Sub-Saharan Africa: The Young of the Future

Sub-Saharan Africa finds itself in a demographic bind of a different sort. Its population is expected to quadruple to 4 billion people by 2100,[44] with Nigeria overtaking America as the world's third most populous country. There is much excitement at the prospect of youth burgeoning as the old world shrinks. Tanzanian President John Magufuli has claimed he sees no need for birth control, insisting a high fertility rate will boost his country's economy.[45]

Sadly, he may be mistaken. The great leaps forward made by the Asian Tiger economies came from the so-called 'demographic dividend': of rapid growth in working-age populations, enabling those countries to grow fast and invest, followed by sharp subsequent falls in the birth rate which boosted the skills base, because parents with fewer children could invest more in educating each one.

Sub-Saharan Africa is on a different path, of continuing population growth with no demographic dividend in sight. Its per capita income is growing slowly, and its many willing hands may not be able to find work, if they remain at low skill levels. Add to that the likely strains on the environment and infrastructure, and Mr Magufuli may come to change his mind.

The Paradox of Living Longer, But Not Being Fertile for Longer

Falling birth rates must be good news for a planet whose natural resources have been stretched to the limit by humans. And they reflect a welcome next step in the liberation of women. Almost everywhere outside sub-Saharan Africa, women are throwing off the shackles of their traditional roles. Lower infant mortality has made it safer to have smaller families. The hold of religion is waning. More women are pursuing careers. At the same time, job insecurity and the high cost of living, especially in cities where the jobs are, has left many couples fearing they can't afford children.

Some worried governments have resorted to bribery. The Polish Ministry of Health put out a terrible video, encouraging the population to 'multiply like rabbits'.[46] Norway, Sweden, Denmark, France, Germany and Russia pay 'baby bonuses'. Some of these schemes have had limited success: France and Sweden have the highest birth rates in Europe. But not all women want to be treated like prize cows. A Danish government video, urging women to 'Do It for Denmark', missed the point: that many women don't want children, and others can't find a good father.

It may be that the post-war baby boom was unusual. Today's combination of greater career opportunities for women, and increased financial pressures, may be returning us to an era when people did not get married, or have children, until they felt they could afford it. Some may leave it too late as a result. Others will feel liberated from the tyrannical view that there is something wrong with you if you're childless.

In Extra Time people study longer, leave home later and may not be settled or solvent until their mid-thirties: when they may hit the hard deadline of the biological clock. That mismatch will leave some couples very disappointed.

For the foreseeable future, it looks as though we will be stuck with male fertility declining from about 45, and female fertility from around 30. In most other respects, though, we remain younger for longer.

2

Younger Than You Thought

The stages of life are changing

MY 19-YEAR-OLD GODDAUGHTER IS looking over my shoulder as I write. Will she be reading this again in 2150, when she will be 150? That is the subject of a $1 billion bet made by two American experts on ageing.

Steven Austad, chair of biology at the University of Alabama at Birmingham, has predicted that there will be a 150-year-old human by the year 2150, based on the many breakthroughs which are slowing ageing in mice (see Chapter 6). His friend Jay Olshansky, public health professor at the University of Illinois, disagrees. He thinks the brain will be an insuperable barrier. 'We can replace hips, hearts and so on, but we can't replace the brain,' he has said.[1]

The two men made the bet in 2000. They each put $150 into an investment fund, and signed a contract certifying that the winner's heirs will cash it out in 2150. They later doubled their initial investment, and now expect the jackpot to be around $1 billion. If Austad is right, someone alive today will still be around to see who wins the bet.

While we wait to see whether lifespans jump to 150, some other changes have already crept up on us. At 19, my goddaughter ought to be emerging from adolescence into adulthood. But she's just started university, is racking up debt and expects to be living with her parents for years to come. So many people are now in this situation, some experts argue that the stage of adolescence should last until 24. That's the average age at which children now move out of the family home in the UK, France, Germany and Australia.

The Australian professor Susan Sawyer has argued that adolescence should be extended in both directions: starting at 10,[2] to reflect the fact that puberty is now starting at that tender age in some girls, and lasting until 24. Extended parental involvement through this later period can be highly beneficial, the psychologist Laurence Steinberg has argued, because we now know that the brain continues to mature into the twenties.

If adolescence now lasts for 14 years, what happens to the subsequent stages of life? They are also lengthening. We saw in the last chapter that people are having children later. Beyond that, mature independent adulthood is lasting longer too.

It's Not Old Age That's Getting Longer, It's Middle Age

Last winter, a doctor friend of mine was in charge of the influenza vaccinations for the over-65s at his local clinic. A crowd of grey-haired strangers walked in. They'd never come to see him before, because there was nothing wrong with them.

These people are part of a growing group who are defying all the labels. They don't see themselves as old, don't act old and won't buy products marketed at the old either.

In England, the proportion of over-65s with any kind of impairment has been falling for two decades.[3] In America, three-quarters of people under 75 have no problems with hearing or vision, no difficulty walking, and no form of cognitive impairment.[4] These are fully fledged citizens with plenty left to offer, not retirees on their way out. Step up a generation, to those aged between 75 and 84, and half still have none of those disabilities.

That doesn't mean that older people don't forget their keys, or lose concentration. But it does mean that some of our fears are overdone. In surveys, most people say they think that everyone will get dementia (or Alzheimer's, a form of dementia) if they live long enough.[5] But only one in six people over 80 have dementia:[6] many never get it. And in Denmark, Sweden,[7] the UK and US, the risk of getting dementia is a fifth lower than it was 20 years ago.[8] In 2000, the average age for receiving a diagnosis of dementia in the US was 80.7; by 2012, it had crept up to 82.4, even though doctors had got better at spotting it.[9]

Experts are not sure why the incidence of dementia is dropping but the Framingham Heart Study, which has tracked 5,000 people over 60, suggests that rates of dementia have mirrored improvements in heart health.[10] In the UK, dementia rates have fallen faster for men than for women, which may be because men previously smoked more. There will still be news headlines about dementia being on the rise but what's growing is the total number of older people, not our own individual risk.

The 'Young-Old': The New Kids on the Block

The Japanese, whose society is now the oldest on the planet, caught up with the reality of Extra Time long ago. The group who are still hale and hearty and rushing around after grandchildren they call the 'Young-Old'. Those who are frail and in need of support they call 'Old-Old'.

'The Young-Old are very active and healthy and productive – totally different from 30 years ago,' says Professor Takao Suzuki, Professor of Gerontology at Tokyo's J F Oberlin University. 'Walking speeds are much faster, for example. The World Health Organization defines "old" as 65, but as gerontologists and geriatricians, our main concern is with the Old-Old, who are very different from a health standpoint.'

Sketching energetically on his whiteboard, Professor Suzuki is, endearingly but disconcertingly, wearing a thin black cowboy tie over his pristine white shirt. He draws a matrix showing the Young-Old starting at 60, and Old-Old from 75 – but says the start date of becoming Old-Old can be much later than that. Professor Suzuki attributes Japan's uniquely long-life expectancy to good medical care, prosperity and improved nutrition after the Second World War, when people could afford to eat far more protein, mostly fish. Consumption of carbohydrates, fat and sugar has barely changed, he says, as fast food outlets are still relatively few. Unlike Western experts, he worries more about under-nourished widows than obesity. (Some widows were not eligible for their husband's full pension, he says, and have trouble getting to the shops to buy groceries.)

The Oldest Stewardess in the World

Bette Nash, 82, is telling me about the time she flew with Jackie Kennedy. It was 1965, and the glamorous wife of the former US president walked onto the flight where Bette was a stewardess. 'We used to have to wear white gloves. I was pulling them on with my back turned and I heard this voice asking, was this flight going to Washington? She was real sweet, never asked for any attention.'

The plane, Bette remembers, was a Constellation – very different to the Airbus she flies now. For Bette Nash is still working. She is probably the oldest stewardess in the world. American Airlines, her employer, recently threw a party to celebrate her 60th anniversary. Regular passengers on the Washington, DC–Boston shuttle bought her gifts.

Bette says she has no intention of retiring: 'I thrive on people.' She talks fast and exudes energy: 'If I'm ever off for a few days and think about stopping, as soon as I get my uniform back on and drive to the airport, it's great. It's the people who work for the airline and it's the customers. I know their little needs. I know the commuter who likes his tomato juice plain in the winter and on ice in the summer. I feel so comfortable going to work.'

Technology has changed in the past 60 years – Bette doesn't have to handwrite the tickets any more – but people haven't changed. 'It's being kind to people, and them being kind to you. A little love and kindness is what everyone needs.'

The job is physically tiring, but Bette makes few concessions: 'If I have free time I don't sit down, I walk the cabin and talk to people. I do have a nap in the afternoon – I'll admit that – but younger people get tired too.' She gets up early in the morning and prepares a meal for her son before driving the hour to the airport. On the way home, she says, she does feel more tired. 'Before, I might have gone to the store on the way home, and done other things; now I might just get gas.'

What is her secret? She pauses. 'When I think about it now, I think my goal in life is to keep moving,' she chuckles. She may sit down to watch TV, but never for long. 'There's always something to do.' She doesn't follow an exercise regime, and admits to eating chocolate, but laughs: 'I can still suck in my tummy.' Almost without knowing it, she seems to have been following three of the tenets of the old-age lifestyle gurus: keep active, retain your sense of purpose and connect with people.

Is Bette Nash old? She thinks for a moment. 'I don't feel like I'm an old person. I have a handicapped son, I don't have the chance to feel old; his needs are so great. My sister has Parkinson's and dementia and I look at her and I think she's old, but she's younger than I am.'

Bette is not 'old' in the way we used to think of it. But her younger sister is. And this is where the debate gets confused. The stereotypes don't fit any more. What we are witnessing is the decoupling of biological age from chronological age.

New Stages Require New Signals

When Otto von Bismarck, the German chancellor, created what was arguably the world's first state pension in 1889, he set the pension age at 70. Few would ever draw it, since the average German lived to around 45.

Today, life expectancy in Germany is 81. But Germany's pension age is 65[11] and the average German gives up work at 62. Right across Europe, retirement ages are not keeping pace with life expectancy. In the UK, men leave the labour force earlier than they did in 1950.[12]

If current trends continue, some of us living in Europe, parts of Asia and North America could spend a quarter of our lives retired. That is crazy.

Lord Adair Turner chaired the independent UK Pensions Commission which recommended in 2005 that the British government should raise the pension age to 66 by 2030, and to 68 by 2050. He now thinks this wasn't sufficiently far-sighted. The UK government now intends to raise the pension age to 67 by 2028, but he thinks 'this won't be nearly enough. In 1950, average male life expectancy at 65 was 12 years. By the time we were looking at it, in 2003, it was 20 years. Life expectancy at 65 could be another 35 years by the time we reach mid-century. We should have started increasing the pension age years before.'

Actuaries, he says, simply didn't realise how fast life expectancy was growing: 'There was a dominant hypothesis about a limit to life. They kept producing curves showing life expectancy growing, but then tailing off. Eventually we said there's no reason to tail off.' Why did they get it so wrong? 'Smoking. The tobacco companies were mass murderers,' says Turner – and no one thought their power would wane.

Pensions are one of many signals which influence how we see older people – and ourselves. These signals need updating.

What it means to be 65 has changed utterly. In the 1950s, a 65-year-old woman in Britain could expect to live a further 14 years.[13] Today, according to the UK's Office for National Statistics, the average 65-year-old woman can look forward a further 23.4 years.[14]

Yet 65 is now the age at which many institutions impose a concept of old age upon their citizens. It's the moment when

Germans, Swedes, Canadians, Australians and Brits can officially retire, and Americans become eligible for full Medicare (federal health insurance). It's a tipping point for financial advisers, who will often start switching your pension portfolio into bonds when you hit your 50s. And '65+' is often the maximum age bracket cited in questionnaires, with no other boxes to tick – as if it's the beginning of the end.

In London, everyone gets a free bus pass when they turn 60. It's called an Older Person's Bus Pass – something which causes a great deal of blushing among the many still-vibrant commuters who could perfectly well afford to pay their own fare. In the US it is entirely normal to call people 'Seniors', and to offer them Senior discounts, for a period of what could, these days, end up being 30 years. Yet much of that period will be spent as Young-Old, not Old-Old.

What if, instead of defining people by how many birthdays they've enjoyed, we define them by how many years they have left? Obviously, that's hypothetical. None of us can know individually when we will meet our end. But we do know the average. And if we apply that average, things look different.

If we defined old age as having 15 years or less left to live, we wouldn't call many baby boomers 'old' until they hit 74. Up to that point they'd be middle-aged. This is a crude measure. Not everyone will be in good health at 74: some will need support. But it's still a useful thought experiment, which has been carried out by a group of demographers at the International Institute for Applied Systems Analysis in Vienna.

The Austrians wanted to challenge the use of 65 as the onset of old age in Europe.[15] First, they ran the numbers for remaining life expectancy. Next, they drew up a list of characteristics which we usually associate with being 'old', such as reduced mental agility and dependency on others. On this basis, across four different countries – Norway, Japan, Lithuania and the US – they concluded most baby boomers remain middle-aged until their mid-seventies.

The insight that chronological age is a poor way to classify who is 'old' came originally from the Canadian-American demographer Norman Ryder, who realised in the 1970s that expected lifespan is a better indicator than age of our need for state support: which is, after all, what the state is interested in.

'If you don't consider people old just because they reached age 65, but instead take into account how long they have left to live, then the faster the increase in life expectancy, the less ageing is actually going on,' explains demographer Sergei Scherbov, leader of the Vienna study. 'Two hundred years ago, a 60-year-old would have been a very old person,' he tells me. 'Someone who is 60 years old today, I would argue, is middle-aged.'

Scherbov is now working with the UN to redesign traditional measures of ageing, using what he calls 'characteristic-equivalent ages'. In 2015, for example, the average Japanese woman of 65 could expect to live another 24 years. But the average woman in Nigeria had to be much younger – 46 – to get 24 more years life expectancy. To be equitable, their pensions would need to start at different ages.

Evolving lifespans should make governments careful about what signals they send, to encourage people to save enough. 'You don't need to tell a 25-year-old when their retirement should be,' says Lord Turner. 'If you tell them there is a fixed retirement age, you are not telling them that things are uncertain. It would be better to tell them, look right now you're in a pension scheme which retires at 65, but that may change with life expectancy.' Lord Turner has suggested making the pension more generous from 70, and means-testing other benefits before that age.[16]

Our Stereotypes Are Out of Date

Institutional signals of this kind are one reason why we have not caught up with the reality of Extra Time. Another is the media. We journalists are deeply confused about age.

In 2018, *The Times* gave a double-page spread to a French lady called Mylène Desclaux,[17] who had published a book about how to be sexy at 50. The breathless article advised women never to give a birthday party after 49, to avoid wearing reading glasses which might give the game away and to change their first name if it sounded too dated. In other words, lie. At 50! What would she suggest women do at 70, I wondered?

If 50 is old to some journalists, 65 is beyond the pale. Sub-editors love to bung 'pensioner' into headlines, making the subject an object of pity no matter what the story. 'Plucky Pensioner Patrols Crime-ridden Streets Armed Only with Torch' was a recent head-line in Cape Town, South Africa. 'Plucky Pensioner Chases Bag Thieves' was another in England's *Swindon Advertiser*, about a 69-year-old who sprinted after a wallet thief. The implication, as usual, was that anyone brave and fit enough to do this at 69 was extraordinary. In fact, the multitude of stories entitled 'plucky pensioner', from all over the world, suggests to me that courage, energy and strength are not uncommon among people who are, in fact, in extended middle age.

The media also has a strange tendency to move from the active to the passive when describing the elderly. 'She had a fall', we report of a grandmother, rather than 'she fell down'. We would never say that of George Clooney. So why do we demean older people in this way? Unconsciously, our language turns people into sub-humans, lesser beings. My mother used to loathe being called 'dear' by strangers: she felt she'd fallen into some void, some category of oldness which robbed her of her identity.

I've fallen into the same trap myself, by focusing on age when it was irrelevant. When I interviewed Margaret Atwood, bestselling Canadian novelist and author of *The Handmaid's Tale*,[18] I asked her how she felt about having 1.6 million followers on Twitter at the age of 77. Atwood, who is one of my heroines, shot back sharply: 'It's 1.75 million!' I felt ashamed. She went on to say, 'A lot of them are robots. You know they are robots when they send you a message saying, "I miss your great big dick".' That was her graceful way of telling me to stop being so bloody patronising. What was I thinking?

'There is a casualness of ageism,' says Professor Martin Green, CEO of Care England. 'People say things they would never say if the word "old" was replaced by "gay" or "black". They say silly old people, shouldn't be driving. But 19-year-olds are worse drivers than 80-year-olds.'

'Everybody ghettoises the old,' says the broadcaster Joan Bakewell. 'But the old is us.' Bakewell, 85, is a poster girl for ageing well. She looks fabulous and has lost none of her sharpness. But when she presented the TV programme *Life at 100* in 2017, she had to keep challenging the production team for referring to older viewers as 'they'. 'There shouldn't be that distinction,' she says. 'We are all in this together.'

Language matters. Baroness Sally Greengross, a formidable campaigner for older people, told me about a friend in her eighties who went to hospital and was admitted to the 'geriatric' ward. 'But I'm not geriatric!' she protested furiously, as they wheeled her away down the corridor. 'Take me somewhere else!'

Women are thought to suffer ageism earlier, and more consistently, than men.[19] That's partly because we care more about how women look. The multi-billion-pound cosmetic industry, with its claim to reverse ageing, may be doing more harm than good. Personally, I see nothing wrong with trying to avoid wrinkles. But advertising does feed off the idea that we are in a constant battle against 'old'. If anti-ageing is becoming synonymous with being anti-old people, we have a problem.

Becca Levy, Associate Professor of Epidemiology and Psychology at the Yale School of Public Health, has found that individuals' own health is influenced by their perceptions of what ageing is like. Her team followed several hundred Americans over 50 for 20 years, and found that those who held more positive views of ageing lived an astonishing 7.5 years longer than their peers.[20]

Negativity is rife. Broadcasters, galleries and museums spend hours worrying about how to reach more youthful audiences – despite the fact that older people have more time and money, and are growing in number. We value youth, tech and energy over wisdom and maturity, or so it seems.

The extreme youth of Silicon Valley plays into all of this. In 2014, the median age of Facebook employees was 29; at Amazon and Google it was 30. Facebook founder Mark Zuckerberg famously quipped, 'Young people are just smarter.' Many of us unthinkingly bought his line – just as we've bought some other lines from Facebook.

The Value of Experience

Chesley 'Sully' Sullenberger was 58 when he safely landed US Airways Flight 1549 in New York's Hudson River after both engines were disabled by a flock of geese, saving everyone on board. The plane juddered across the Manhattan skyline and plunged safely into the icy water between the narrow banks. It was an extraordinary feat, which was turned into a Hollywood movie – *Sully* (2016) – by Clint Eastwood.

'One way of looking at this,' Sully reflected afterwards, 'might be that for 42 years, I've been making small, regular deposits in this bank of experience, education and training. And on January 15, the balance was sufficient so that I could make a very large withdrawal.'

That wonderfully modest, laconic statement sums up the value of cumulative expertise. I'm not claiming that every 58-year-old is a hero-in-the-making – and I've seen good ideas from young people being ignored because they are not considered mature enough – but I do feel that we live in a world more interested in 'digital skills' than judgement, which only comes with experience. Personally, I don't want to be flown by a novice pilot any more than I want to be operated on by a surgeon still in training. I want the guy who's done the same procedure a thousand times.

Some economists believe that ageing workforces are behind the decline in Western productivity. But what if part of the problem is that baby boomers are retiring in droves, taking with them valuable experience and institutional memory?

'I am of the old school,' said English barrister Jerry Hayes, 64, describing how he intervened to save an innocent young man from being jailed for rape.[21] Hayes was supposed to be prosecuting the man, but his 40 years of experience at the English Bar made 'alarm bells ring' when he took over the case at the eleventh hour and asked a police officer whether there were any mobile-phone messages from the man's accuser. The officer insisted he hadn't bothered to show the messages to the defence as there was nothing in them, but Hayes stood his ground and demanded the evidence. 40,000 messages were then handed over, which showed that the so-called 'victim' had been pestering the man continually for sex. The case collapsed and a terrible miscarriage of justice was avoided – but only because of the intuition, experience and sheer bloody-mindedness of a man with a white beard who believed that getting justice was more important than nailing up another successful prosecution.

How Much Extra Time Might *You* Get?

To get an idea of your life expectancy, type a few facts about yourself into an online pension calculator. Let's say you tell it you are a healthy white Englishman, born in 1958. The calculator will give you a life expectancy of 90.

That may come as a shock. Most of us massively underestimate how long we have to live. We tend to think 'when did Granny die?'

rather than realising that we have gained Extra Time. People in their fifties and sixties underestimate their chances of survival to age 75 by 20 per cent according to the UK Institute for Fiscal Studies. Widows and widowers are especially pessimistic.

None of us likes to think about death. But if we fear it's around the corner when it isn't, there's a risk we may start to feel 'old' too soon. We won't save enough, plan our career far enough ahead, or, frankly, feel positive enough about our future.

Of course, averages don't tell us much about our own individual prospects. Our longevity can be boosted by all sorts of things: our income, fitness, even whether we are married or not (married people live longer). But the single most powerful predictor of how long each of us will live turns out to be our level of education. The more time you spent in education in early life, the more Extra Time you are likely to have at the end. And the better your chances of spending that Extra Time in good health.

The figures are surprising. In 2008, white American men with one or more degrees were expected to live up to *14 years longer* than black American men who didn't finish high school.[22] In OECD countries, the gap between men with those education levels is around 7 years.[23]

Education is a stronger predictor of lifespan than wealth. Well-educated Cuba, though dirt poor, has higher life expectancies than America. Oil-rich but poorly educated Equatorial Guinea, on the other hand, has low average life expectancies. So stark are these differences, one expert has suggested that governments should invest more in schools than in hospitals.[24]

The Geography of Life Chances

I'm standing outside the Abbey Road Studios in London's St John's Wood. This is where The Beatles recorded some of their greatest hits and the traffic has stopped as four French tourists attempt to re-create the Fab Four's famous *Abbey Road* album cover, by walking across the black-and-white zebra crossing. I cycle past here regularly, and I know that every tourist imagines they were the first to have the idea. A taxi driver gives me a weary look.

From Abbey Road, a prosperous area in the Borough of Westminster with red-brick mansion blocks and detached houses, I'm cycling south to meet a friend for coffee. I'm going to do a route I take often, along backstreets. What I didn't know, until recently, was that this route spans 10 years of life expectancy.[25]

At Abbey Road, female life expectancy at birth is around 87 years and 85 for men. I cycle south, towards Lord's cricket ground, into Church Street ward. Here, female life expectancy has dropped to 81 years and it's 80 for men. I make a right turn towards St Mary's Hospital, Paddington, where I was born, and cut along the canal to Westbourne Park tube station, where I'm meeting my friend. By now, female life expectancy has dropped to 77 years and to 75 for men. In a 15-minute trip, life expectancy has changed by a decade. A baby girl who is born and who lives her life in Abbey Road can expect to live, on average, 10 years longer than one born just 1.5 miles away.

You can find similar gaps in many Western regions. Raj Chetty of Stanford University has found a 15-year gap in lifespan between the poorest and richest Americans. But he has also found that absolute income seems to matter less than where you live. The poorest live five years longer in New York and Los Angeles than they do in Tulsa and Detroit. In those areas, Chetty's work suggests that smoking, drinking, stress and obesity have more impact on lifespan than income inequality or unemployment, although of course the two are linked.

Are You Heading for a Nursing Home, or the Beach?

'In the end,' as Abraham Lincoln said, 'it is not the years in your life that count. It is the life in your years.' In surveys, people say repeatedly that they don't want to live to 100 if that means spending their last years in some ghostly half-life of senescence.

In the twentieth century, when most of us died from infectious diseases, increases in life expectancy generally implied an improvement in health for everybody. In the twenty-first century, that link has broken. Longevity is bringing some people more years of good health, but others more years of frailty.

There are two reasons for this. First, medical advances mean that things which used to kill us, like heart attacks and stroke, are less often fatal. We can keep people alive, stumbling gratefully on, some in good shape, others less so. Second, there has been an explosion in chronic conditions, like type 2 diabetes, high blood pressure, dementia and respiratory disease, which are often linked to smoking, drinking and lack of physical activity.

Differences in those behaviours are one reason why people living in the South East of England, for example, are likely to enjoy eight more years of life free from disability than those who live in the North East, according to the Newcastle epidemiologist Carol Jagger.[26]

To get a handle on all of this, statisticians have started to track not only life expectancy but 'healthy life expectancy', defined as the years spent in 'very good' or 'good' health, and 'disability-free life expectancy': the years spent without any limiting condition. The methodology is not terribly robust as it's all based on surveys people fill in, reporting how they feel. The categories are broad too: being in 'poor health' could mean that you suffer from arthritis and can't walk as far as you used to, or that you have early stage dementia. There's an urgent need for better data. But even so, the patterns are striking.

From as young as 40, some less-educated people report having a 'functional limitation' in walking, driving, or some other aspect of daily life. By the age of 60, graduates are in significantly better health than non-graduates. At 85, over half of graduates are still living happily, with no functional limitation.[27] We will see in Chapter 5 that some highly educated people also seem to have 'cognitive reserve', which can be protective against Alzheimer's.

It is not clear exactly why education is so vital. Some experts argue that education is formative. It may make us better at planning, and exercising self-control, which may feed into healthier lifestyle choices. It also affects the kind of jobs we do. Lower-skilled jobs can be physically taxing, emotionally stressful and – it turns out – bad for health.

The legendary Whitehall II Study of British civil servants,[28] led by the epidemiologist Sir Michael Marmot in the early 2000s, found that staff doing the lowest skilled jobs, like messengers and door-keepers, had a mortality rate *three times higher* than permanent secretaries and top managers. They also had far higher levels of corti-sol, the stress hormone associated with coronary heart disease.[29] Marmot's findings may seem counter-intuitive, but they make sense. Senior executives may work longer hours and face gruelling deci-sions, but support staff have lower social status, far less control over their working environment and probably a longer commute.

Life has never been fair. But as we live longer, less-educated and poorer people are becoming 'Old-Old' earlier than richer and more educated ones, and the gap is widening.[30] Professor James Nazroo, at the University of Manchester, has found that when they turn 80, the richest third of Britons is only just beginning to experience the limit-ations that people in the poorest third have been suffering from 70.

Narrowing that gap, providing people with more equal life chances, must surely be one of the most important social justice missions of our times. The rich and well educated already know some of the secrets to making the most of Extra Time – and there are more in this book. But unless we spread that knowledge to everyone, we will all be the poorer.

One country is leading the way. The Japanese government has set itself an explicit aim of 'extending Healthy Life Expectancy more than the increase of Average Life Expectancy' through its Health Japan 21 initiative.[31] Ministers are working to actively combat what they call 'lifestyle-related diseases' with detailed targets for everything from salt intake to blood pressure levels, to the number of steps people take every day. Different provinces run programmes encouraging people to stay fit, reduce their smoking and drinking, and to take care of themselves.

These schemes are getting traction. The average Japanese man gained an entire extra year of healthy life between 2013 and 2016 (women gained six months).[32] This was a win for Extra Time, since life expectancy at birth rose by nine months for men and six months for women in the same period.[33]

These schemes build on the strong Japanese tradition of self-reliance. Many Japanese people I have interviewed do not want to be a burden to their children as they age, nor do they expect the state to do everything. They are willing to try and ditch bad habits. If other countries emulate this approach, tackling behaviour throughout the life course, not just at the beginning or the end, we might close the gap.

You're Only as Old as You Feel

Spring Chicken, a British start-up which sells home gadgets to the elderly, conducted a survey which asked: 'What age do you feel – on the outside, and on the inside?'[34] Most people between 50 and 90 reported feeling a few years younger than their actual age on the outside, but considerably younger on the inside. The older the respondents, the bigger the gap. Eighty-year-olds in the survey reported that they felt about 50 years old on the inside. Are they delusional, or might they just be on to something?

'People will say things like, "I still feel 30, it's just my knees are letting me down,"' says Anna James, who founded the business after a fruitless and frustrating search for gadgets to help her father, who is 74 and has Parkinson's. Her father now works in her business and tests out products, yet even he refuses to see himself as needing help. In 2017, James realised her father was getting to the point where he was going to need an electric wheelchair, but he wouldn't consider it. 'You've got to battle with the psyche,' she says. So she asked him to test out electric wheelchairs and write a blog about his favourite model. Eventually, the time came. 'Could I borrow that wheelchair for a few weeks?' he asked. 'He took it on a cruise with my mother,' she says, 'and ended up selling one to another guest on board!' This was a man who was still young and dynamic inside – and able to make a sale.

Reasons to Be Cheerful

Extra Time has given us an entirely new stage of life: the stage of the 'Young-Old'. We need to catch up with this new reality, stop lumping everyone from 60 to 100 together, and accept that it is normal to be vibrant and capable in your seventies. Media editors should take a look at how they portray 'pensioners', and question whether they are falling for a narrow narrative about youth. Governments must raise retirement ages in line with life expectancy and make this explicit: as part of signalling that the average lifespan has changed. And all of us need to challenge our own attitudes. Prejudices we build up against the 'old' will only hurt us when we reach that stage ourselves.

One vital question is what proportion of the over-60s will be 'Young-Old', thriving and capable like stewardess Bette Nash, and how many will be 'Old-Old', needing care, like her sister. On the answer to that question rests the future of our economies and the cohesion of our societies. If there are too many 'Old-Old', our welfare states and healthcare systems will be overloaded and younger generations will bear the burden. But if we can help people to stay healthy and productive, if we can abolish prejudice, we could see a new era of extended middle age, with most people staying vital almost to the end.

Later in this book I describe breakthroughs in genetics and neuroscience which may transform the youthspan, elongating our 'Young-Old' period and limiting the 'Old-Old'. But we don't have to wait for those. We already hold two of the keys in our hands to improving our Extra Time: diet and exercise.

3

Just Do It

If exercise and diet was a pill, we'd all be taking it

WHAT IF THE KIND of ageing we dread is not, in fact, normal? What if our modern accumulation of chronic diseases, followed by a prolonged twilight zone, are largely a consequence of Western habits, which have distorted the true path of biological ageing?

It's generally assumed that how we age is down to luck and genetic inheritance. But for most of us, genes write only 20 per cent of our fate. The other 80 per cent is down to environmental factors: what we eat and drink, how stressful our lives are, whether we live amid pollution, whether we exercise (and how often).

This means that we already hold many of the keys to Extra Time in our own hands. Decades of research show that we don't have to succumb to deterioration from the age of 50, our arteries and joints gradually stiffening, and puffing our way into chronic disease. We can fight to stay relatively youthful right up until 90, and even reduce our risk of dementia, by eating better and becoming far, far more active. A raft of studies around the world have, in fact, identified exercise as the single most powerful predictor of whether we will age well.[1]

'Miracle Cure', a report from the Academy of Medical Royal Colleges, finds that the big four 'proximate' causes of preventable ill health are smoking, poor nutrition, lack of physical activity and alcohol excess. 'Of these,' the report says, 'the importance of regular exercise is the least well-known. But relatively low levels of increased activity can make a huge difference'. The report concluded that 30 minutes of moderately intense exercise, five times a week, can reduce the risk of developing heart disease, stroke, type 2 diabetes, some cancers and even dementia.[2]

This needs to be much, much better-known.

If Life Is a Marathon, We Need to Sprint

'If exercise was a pill, everyone would be taking it,' says Norman Lazarus, 82, as we walk through a violent downpour outside his office at London Bridge. My feet are drenched even under my umbrella; he only has a jaunty red cap on his head, but he shrugs off the rain. A short, wiry man with a stubby white moustache, Lazarus is a long-distance cyclist who regularly covers distances of 60 miles. He has just come back from cycling 180 miles in Oxfordshire with his daughter at the weekend. 'Exercise is great,' he says, in his strong South African accent. 'For the body, the mind, for muscles – you name it.'

Lazarus is not just a biking fanatic, he is also emeritus professor at King's College London, where he has co-authored a study into amateur endurance cyclists like himself. The older cyclists in the study – aged between 55 and 79 – were found to have similar immune systems, strength, muscle mass and cholesterol levels as those who were only in their twenties.[3] On those criteria, the older cyclists had barely aged at all. The researchers could not tell how old they were by looking at their physiology on paper, only by meeting them and seeing their wrinkles.

The King's researchers believe that endurance sports, including cycling, swimming and running, may protect the immune system by boosting the number of T-cells in our blood. These protective white blood cells are thought to decline by about 2 per cent a year from our twenties onwards, making us gradually more susceptible to infections and conditions like rheumatoid arthritis. But the older endurance cyclists had almost as many T-cells as 20-year-olds – a protective effect that no medicine yet invented can provide.

To qualify for the study, men had to be able to cycle 62 miles in under 6.5 hours and women had to be able to cycle 37 miles in 5.5 hours. That's impressive. But all were amateurs, not professionals. Some, like Norman Lazarus, had only taken up cycling in their fifties. And they loved it. When interviewed, they reported not only managing the distances fine, but feeling fabulous as a result and wanting to do more.

Lazarus cycles with an amateur group. He also goes to the gym three times a week and does what he calls 'anti-gravity exercises' – lifting weights. Many of his friends cycle, as does his wife, who is 85. 'We're all going to die, yes,' he announces breezily, 'but none of us are ill at the moment. One day we'll get to the point where we can no longer fight infection. But then hopefully, it will be quick' – he pulls his hands towards each other to demonstrate the narrowing period of illness, the mercifully brief end he anticipates when he and his friends eventually move from 'Young-Old' to 'Old-Old'.

Do the cyclists keep going because they are unusually healthy, or are they healthy because they cycle? Lazarus believes it's the latter. What we see in the cyclists, he insists, 'is true biological ageing, free from the problems caused by inactivity'.

If you wanted to see what true biological ageing might look like, you could charter a boat. In Ikaria, a beautiful Greek island off the west coast of Turkey, one in three inhabitants live into their nineties and dementia is rare. Ikarian men don't get cancer or heart disease very often, and when they do, it develops eight to ten years later than in Americans. Ikarians also report considerably less depression.[4] Their life is very much an outdoor one – it's said to be hard to get through a day in Ikaria without walking up 20 hills – and that might just have something to do with it.

Ikaria is one of the Blue Zones (see page 4), where people live exceptionally long lives in good health. There doesn't seem to be any genetic singularity; the secret is lifestyle. There has been much talk about the plant-based diets eaten in Blue Zones and far less focus on exercise. But whether in Sardinia, Okinawa or the other

Blue Zones, it's clear that these hearty, long-lived people lead very active outdoor lives.

This is not 'exercise' in a gym, pumping iron to music videos. It's movement built into daily life, to do tasks that the rest of us have replaced with cars, robot-vacuum cleaners and other devices. We have saved ourselves hours by not fetching water, chopping wood or tending our vegetables. But has it lost us our agility? Activity maintains muscle mass, reduces stress by connecting our primitive brain to its old hunter-gathering functions and improves immunity by triggering a cascade of chemical signals in the body. Whenever we take the lift rather than the stairs, or drive rather than walk, we may be losing more than we realise.

Until now I've thought of endurance athletes as freakish, as having either a genetic predisposition or a crazy obsession to compete. But now I wonder. Stunning results have been seen in an otherwise normal group of American septuagenarians who started running when it became fashionable during the 1970s, and stayed hooked. Over the next 50 years some went on jogging, others took up cycling or swimming or working out, but they did it regularly – and as a hobby, not to compete.

To the amazement of the researchers, the muscle strength of these seventy-somethings was almost indistinguishable from 25-year-olds, with as many capillaries and enzymes. Their aerobic capacity was 40 per cent higher than people of their age who were not regular exercisers. The researchers at Ball State University, Indiana, concluded this made both the men and the women biologically *30 years younger* than their chronological age.[5]

It's impossible to overstate the importance of this finding: it suggests there is hope for us all.

Younger Next Year?

In terms of fitness, human beings keep pushing the boundaries of what is thought possible. The 'Masters' sporting events are a kind of

amateur Olympics for those aged between 35 and 100. These regularly generate headlines about extraordinary feats – like in 2016,
when Japanese athlete Hiroo Tanaka ran the 100 metres in 15.19
seconds. Tanaka's time was nowhere near the Jamaican Usain Bolt's
world record-setting run of 9.58 seconds in the final of the 2009
World Athletics Championships in Berlin. But Bolt was 23, Tanaka
was 85.

Masters athletes don't just sustain performance to advanced ages,
they have also been improving constantly over time. Their athletic
performance has improved 'significantly and progressively' in the
past 40 years. And the greatest magnitude of improvements has been
made by the oldest swimmers and runners, who are over 75.[6] This
suggests that we may be only in the foothills of understanding the
'Young-Old'. One of the Holy Grails for serious sportspeople – the
maximal rate of oxygen consumption or VO_2 max – declines at half
the rate in Masters athletes as it does in their sedentary peers.[7] One
explanation is that regular aerobic exercise brings more oxygen to
the muscles. The more we do, the more our heart and circulation
respond, to get oxygen round the body.

Intensive working out doesn't massively extend life. Olympians gain
only 3 extra years over normal folk on average, according to a century
of Games records.[8] But they do gain a significant health advantage.
This is greatest for cyclists and rowers, apparently; but even playing
lower-intensity sports like golf can be positive. Commenting on the
research, Professors Adrian Bauman of Sydney University and Steven
Blair of South Carolina University stressed we don't all have to be
Olympic athletes to reap the benefits of exercise and win a 'personal
gold medal'. They urged governments to do far more to improve physical activity.

We don't all have to run marathons. Above a certain level of
athleticism, you can't advance your health, only your performance.
'Think back over 40,000 years of evolution,' says Norman Lazarus.
'We had to be fit to hunt. But you wouldn't chase an animal for 15

miles – that wouldn't be worth it, just to get, say, a pound of steak. You'd stop after a mile and keep tracking.'

That's a relief. I don't enjoy running – I can only sustain it with friends, shuffling through corny hits on my headphones. But Lazarus does make me wonder how many of us modern office workers would have the stamina to track our prey for miles, if we were suddenly transported to a desert plain. Nervously, I ask whether he thinks I am doing enough. I do British Military Fitness twice a week in my local park, cycle to meetings if I can and play a slow game of tennis once a week. I don't mention that I achieve this only on good weeks. 'Perfect,' he beams, as if I have made it into a club. 'Do what you enjoy.' He pauses. 'But' – he fixes me with a glare – 'your goals do need to be sufficiently ambitious.'

Ambition is frankly what most of us lack. When I started research-ing this book, I thought I was pretty fit. Now, I realise with horror that I've slumped into a rather comfy regime. My tennis game is doubles, not singles, and includes gossip and cappuccino. I've dropped into the slow group at Military Fitness. I don't work up a sweat as often as I used to. And what many experts seem to believe, though few dare to put it so crudely, is that sweat is the measure which really matters.

Ambitious is also what our health systems are not. Older people are so often told: 'don't overdo it'. Yet from the age of 50, muscle and bone mass start to decline by around 2 per cent a year.[9] We should be doubling down on strength training and aerobic fitness from that age. Instead, we spend an awful lot of time sitting down: something we are now told is as dangerous as smoking.

Don't Just Sit There – Do Something

The idea that sitting is as dangerous as smoking sounds absurd, but evidence from all over the world, from Norway to Canada, suggests a lack of low-level physical activity is cumulatively crippling. It puts us at much greater risk of getting the same nasty diseases which exercise can help to prevent.[10] That doesn't mean it's your fault if you get cancer: I abhor the invidious trend which implies that people who fall sick didn't do enough sit-ups or eat enough broccoli. But so compelling is the evidence, I predict that in 20 years' time it will seem as foolish not to exercise every day as it does now to keep smoking.

We've known that sedentary occupations were dangerous since 1953, when J. N. Norris and colleagues reported in *The Lancet* that London bus drivers were more likely to suffer heart disease than London bus conductors.[11] This was a brilliantly elegant piece of research. The two groups of staff worked the same hours, breathed the same air and hailed from similar backgrounds. The main difference was that the drivers were sitting down all day, the conductors were moving around taking tickets and chatting to people. Without knowing it, the conductors had chosen a far healthier job.

Sitting down for more than an hour at a time sharply decreases the enzyme LPL, which burns body fat and produces good cholesterol.[12] It can also weaken leg and hip muscles, which makes older people more likely to fall. A weekend workout will not erase the effect of prolonged hours sitting in our cars, at our desks or at a screen. In the US and UK, only a quarter of us are apparently moving around enough during the working day, and in Australia, only a third. Older adults have the lowest levels of physical activity, with only 7 per cent of Brits achieving the recommended minimum of five times a week.[13]

It's not easy to improve, especially if you earn your living driving a truck or typing. Fitbits may help: people who take 10,000 steps a day apparently have lower blood pressure, more stable glucose levels and better moods than those who don't.[14] There's no special magic to the 10,000 target – it apparently derives from the first pedometers sold by a Japanese company in the 1960s, which were called *manpo-kei*, or '10,000-step meter'. Some people think 15,000 steps better resemble the daily distances covered by the average Ikarian or Okinawan, but the point is to keep trying, every day.

Could What We Think of as 'Ageing' Actually Be Lack of Fitness?

'We have a muddled concept of ageing,' says Sir Muir Gray, Clinical Advisor to Public Health England, former Chief of Knowledge for the NHS, and author of the wonderfully named book *Sod 70!* 'Society perceives disease, loss of fitness, dependency, dementia and frailty as inevitable,' he says. 'But they are not.'

With a shock of white hair at 73, and a wiry energy, Gray clearly has no intention of slowing down. He arrives sporting a pair of black Nike trainers and announces in his rasping Scottish brogue that he has walked to our meeting – I dare not ask how far since it may put me to shame. Gray is passionately convinced that we confuse the effects of true ageing with what is mainly a loss of fitness, caused by far too little activity. 'People with long-term conditions and those who experience pain,' he says, 'often mistakenly believe that exercise will make things worse, rather than understanding that the more conditions you have, the more you need to improve the four aspects of fitness: strength, stamina, suppleness and skill.' Some doctors prescribe exercise – for osteoarthritis, for example – but not for many other conditions.

Gray believes we could save billions if we made it normal to expect people of all ages to be active. 'Almost every week, there are headlines about the rising cost of health and social care,' he explains. 'The blame is usually placed on the rising numbers of older people, as if the requirement for social care was an unavoidable consequence of ageing. But exercise can reduce the need for social care.' In 2017, he and colleagues calculated that the UK could save several billions a year from 'even modest improvements in fitness' to stop older people crossing the line from independence to dependence: needing carers or going into a home.[15]

Unless we are rigorous about keeping active, natural decline will be accelerated by unnatural stiffness, extra loss of muscle tone and immunity, and hardening of the arteries. Gray calls this the 'fitness gap', which opens up between how able we are and how able we could be. This starts, imperceptibly, in our thirties. By our sixties, we may find we cannot do the basic things we want to do: run for a bus or climb the stairs, for example. If we don't heed the warnings, we may end up crossing the line into dependency.

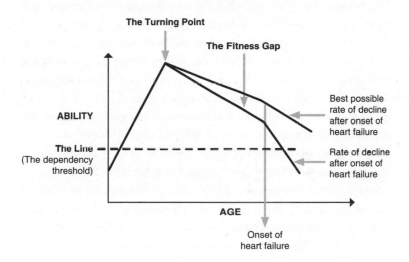

The fitness gap can be narrowed, Gray argues, from any age. Even 90-year-olds can improve their strength with relatively small amounts of exercise.[16] Three months of balance and gait training, and mild weight-bearing exercises, can reduce falls – which are responsible for five times as many hospitalisations among the over-65s as any other injury. They can make the difference between whether someone remains independent, or crosses the line into dependency on others.

In the UK, 10 per cent of ambulances are called out for older people who have fallen over.[17] Half of those who fracture a hip subsequently become reliant on others. Yet physical activity can halve the risk of falls.[18] It also strengthens muscle and bone density, making fractures less likely.[19] From a cost–benefit point of view, let alone a humanitarian standpoint, we should be investing in such programmes in every community.

A little bit of imagination would go a long way here. One company, MIRA Rehab, is using gaming software to improve balance in people aged 3 to 102. In one game, you play a piano by sitting down or standing up: each movement sounds a different key. One stroke victim was so keen to play the whole tune, says MIRA's founder Cosmin Mihaiu, that he managed to sit down and stand up more times than his therapist had imagined possible. A trial has found statistically significant improvements in balance and pain among people who played the games 3 times a week for 12 weeks.[20]

Yet many 90-year-olds who want to exercise come up against the prevailing attitude that exercise is for young people and that older people should relax. We give people pills to stave off pain rather than prescribe exercise which might resolve it. In England, everyone over 60 gets prescription medicines for free. Ontario, Canada, has just followed suit by eliminating the cost of prescription drugs for many senior citizens.[21] But gym memberships aren't free, nor is physiotherapy. Instead of encouraging people to take responsibility for their own health, helping them to understand their bodies and strengthen their muscles, we are making it easiest to pop a pill. That sends the wrong message.

If we were serious about keeping people from crossing the line to dependency, we would put huge effort not only into preventing falls, but also delaying the onset of dementia. Much of the focus has been on finding a cure, which as yet shows no signs of success. But if we could delay onset in individuals by only five years, we would reduce the number of cases by a third. That's because dementia is a disease which usually hits late in life.[22]

The 2,500 Welshmen Who Showed How to Stave Off Dementia

In 1979, an eager young scientist called Peter Elwood trudged up and down the streets of Caerphilly, a valley town in South Wales, knocking on doors. He and his team asked every man between the ages of 45 and 59 if they would let themselves be poked, prodded and interviewed by medics every five years to track their health.

They must have been very persuasive because they got 90 per cent of the candidates – 2,500 Welshmen – to agree.

Caerphilly is set in stunning countryside and is home to one of the greatest medieval castles in Europe, but it's not a rich area. Elwood picked it, unromantically, because there was a high incidence of heart disease.[23] Elwood had been a part of the team which proved that aspirin could protect against heart disease and he was hoping to find a test which would show who would benefit from aspirin most. He failed to do that, but over the next 35 years of the study he discovered something with even greater ramifications.

When I first read about the Caerphilly Cohort Study, it blew me away. I couldn't believe that I'd never heard of it before. For it suggests that making simple lifestyle changes can dramatically lower the risk of cancer, diabetes, heart attack, stroke and even dementia.

The researchers took blood samples, weighed each man and asked five simple questions. Was he a non-smoker? Did he take exercise, or walk, for at least 30 minutes a day, five days a week? Did his diet include at least three portions of fruit and vegetables a day and no more than 30 per cent fat? Did he drink less than four units of alcohol a day? And did he have a healthy body weight (a BMI of 18 to 25)?

Over the next 35 years, men who consistently answered yes to four or five of those questions had a staggeringly better quality of life than those who didn't.[24] They suffered 70 per cent less from diabetes, had 60 per cent fewer heart attacks and strokes, 35 per cent less cancer[25] and were 60 per cent less likely to experience cognitive impairment or dementia. Elwood called this last finding 'the real gold dust'. Even those in the healthiest groups who did get dementia got it later: its onset was delayed by six to seven years.

Remember, these results were achieved with relatively minimal change. The team wasn't asking people to become cycling fanatics, only to start walking and cut down drinking and smoking. They even lowered the diet criteria from five vegetables or fruit a day to three after they were advised that there was no hope of getting anyone in South Wales to eat five!

'From the results in Caerphilly,' Elwood has said, 'we can make a very strong challenge that if every person was urged to take up one extra healthy behaviour, and if only half did so, we'd see 12 per cent less diabetes, 6 per cent fewer heart attacks and strokes and 13 per cent less people with dementia. There would be savings in the NHS of millions.'

Those savings, however, have never materialised. Relatively few men in Elwood's study managed to stick to four of the healthy behaviours. Thirty-five years later, looking back on his life's work, Elwood reflected that behaviours in that part of Wales had changed little.[26] 'We have found that living a healthy lifestyle is better than any pill,' he said in 2013. But 'people are not motivated'.

This must change. For Elwood's findings on dementia have been reinforced by subsequent studies. In 2017, the Lancet Commission on Dementia stated, 'there is evidence that an important fraction of dementia is preventable' through tackling diabetes, obesity, high blood pressure, physical inactivity and smoking.[27]

Food as Medicine

In 2017, the Finnish Geriatric Intervention Study to Prevent Cognitive Impairment and Disability (which has the marvellous acronym FINGER)[28] reported even more encouraging findings about the effects of lifestyle changes on the brain. Researchers recruited 1,260 people aged between 60 and 77, who were judged to be at increased risk of dementia. Half received regular health advice, the other half a comprehensive programme of healthy eating, strength training, aerobic exercise and brain training (which we will look at in Chapter 6). After two years, those who had eaten better, got more active and trained their brains scored 25 per cent better in memory and mental tests than the first group. Even more incredibly, they experienced an 83 per cent improvement in executive functioning and 150 per cent increase in mental processing speed. Intriguingly, these improvements occurred regardless of gender, education level, socioeconomic status, blood pressure or cholesterol levels.

Diet was a key part of FINGER. At the start of the study, participants deemed to be overweight were advised to lose between 5 and 10 per cent of their body weight by reducing the number of calories they consumed. Next, they were instructed to eat lots of fruit and vegetables, to consume fish at least twice a week, to choose wholegrain cereal products over refined ones and to use vegetable margarine or rapeseed oil instead of butter. They were also asked to limit their sugar intake to a maximum of 50g per day and to limit rich dairy and meat foods.

This kind of 'Nordic' or 'Mediterranean' style diet broadly reflects the plant-based, high-fibre food consumed in the Blue Zones. These diets are achievable for middle-income people without having to visit bizarre shops or spend a fortune on the latest fad.

Embarking on regimes which make you feel like a failure is just discouraging but a good basic rule is that what's good for the heart is generally good for the brain. That means eating oodles of vegetables and fruit, plenty of fibre and avoiding processed foods as much as possible. It also means trying to eat in moderation and burn more calories than we consume.

The problem is that these messages aren't landing. The Lancet Commission forecasts that increasing mid-life rates of obesity will lead to a 19 per cent increase in dementia in China and a 9 per cent increase in the US by 2030.[29] That is tragic.

We Are Our Own Worst Enemies

Professor Andrea Maier, geriatrician at the University of Melbourne, Australia, has put it wonderfully bluntly: 'We are very lazy, we are a very lazy species and we just have to overcome that.' She states there are three main reasons why two people can look very different from each other at the age of 50. These are: first, their levels of physical activity; second, whether they smoke; and third, their diet.

Smoking rates are falling, of course. But even as we are vanquishing smoking, obesity is rising to take its place.

My mother could have drawn the chart below. A chain smoker from the age of 14, she took up cigarettes as an act of rebellion at her American convent school. She didn't give up until she was 70, when her arteries got so clogged that she had a mini stroke. It was a dreadful struggle for her to give up cigarettes, even with the help of nicotine patches. She immediately began gorging on chocolate, put on two stone and lost the perfect figure of which she'd been so proud. She became diabetic and later developed vascular

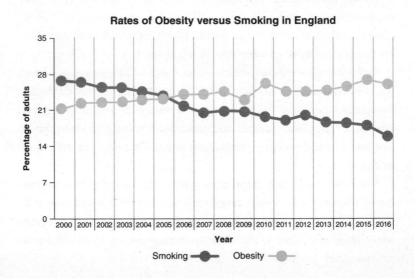

Rates of Obesity versus Smoking in England

dementia. I couldn't help thinking, after her final, fatal heart attack, that she might have been happier staying on the fags. She existed almost entirely on ready meals after she left my father – she said she never wanted to cook for anyone again. And she never took any exercise: for most of her generation it was simply not on their horizon.

To start with, my mother didn't really notice what was happening. As it becomes normal to be fat, people who see others the same size as them may not even notice. The psychological tendency to 'anchor' to those around us is very strong: in one study of 3,000 parents, a third did not even recognise that their own children were obese or overweight.[30]

A vociferous lobby insists that obesity is genetic, but my mother came from a line of beanpoles. Look at any map showing the spread of the disease. It's simply not possible that an epidemic like this could be genetic, eating its way through every US state, English counties and regions of Mexico. Genes do 'load the gun', making some people struggle harder to resist food and to manage their weight. But it is environment – diet and sedentary lifestyles – which 'pulls the trigger'.

One in four adults in the UK, and four in ten in the US, are now clinically obese. Britons have the highest average body mass index in Western Europe.[31] That's because we are eating more calories than we burn. The average American's total calorie intake grew from 2,109 calories in 1970 to 2,568 calories in 2010[32] – the equivalent of eating an extra steak sandwich every day. Few people are exercising enough to compensate, especially as they drive more.

Some experts now think diet is actually less important than car ownership. In 1949, 34 per cent of miles in the UK travelled using a mechanical mode were made by bicycle; today, only 1–2 per cent are.[33] There is a stunning correlation between driving more miles and getting fatter – with a six-year time lag.[34]

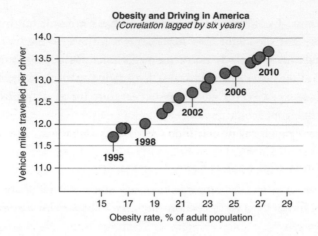

Obesity and Driving in America
(Correlation lagged by six years)

Obesity Is Making People Old Before Their Time

Extreme obesity can knock eight years off your life, according to one Canadian study. But even being overweight has a clear impact on how we age. One study found that obese people had substantially less white matter in their brains than leaner people. While our brains naturally shrink with age, the brains of the obese people were found to have a comparable white matter volume to a lean person 10 years their senior.[35] The impact on cognitive function is not known, but it's unlikely to be good.

Obesity is the main cause of type 2 diabetes, which is most prevalent in older people. The number of Brits with type 2 diabetes has doubled in 20 years[36] and it now accounts for almost 9 per cent of the annual NHS budget. A third of Americans over 65 now have type 2 diabetes.[37] The consequences can be really nasty: blurred vision, sores which won't heal, even toe, foot and leg amputations.

Type 2 diabetes develops when our bodies consume so many carbohydrates that the pancreas ceases to release the right amounts of the hormone insulin into the blood, to regulate the glucose that gives us energy. Our systems are overwhelmed and they fail.

People who head into their sixties obese are storing up real trouble in Extra Time. Doctors are wary of interfering, because they feel that what we eat is a 'lifestyle choice'. Personally, I'm not so sure how much of a choice it is. Public health agencies have spent decades exhorting people to lose weight with almost no effect. I have become convinced that one reason we find it so hard to lose weight is that junk food – especially sugar – is addictive.

The Story of the Sugar Tax

When I served on the board of the Care Quality Commission, the national regulator for hospitals, the scourge of obesity was everywhere. Hospitals were having to reinforce beds for super-sized patients. Doctors were refusing knee replacements to people who were so overweight they feared the replacements would buckle under the strain. Some of those people became less active because their joints hurt and so gained even more weight. It was a terrible vicious cycle.

Around the same time I watched a talk by the American paediatric endocrinologist Professor Robert Lustig.[38] He argues that sugar is the main cause of obesity, because sugar is as addictive as nicotine and switches on the same hormonal pathways which reward behaviour. Low blood sugar affects mood, concentration and the ability to inhibit impulse. Eating or drinking something sugary reverses the effect, but if the pattern is repeated for long enough, it results in insulin resistance, type 2 diabetes, heart disease and obesity. Professor Lustig believes that it is not possible for most people to quit through willpower because that has been eroded by the cycle of craving.

My mother's switch from nicotine to sugar made Lustig's narrative especially compelling for me: she simply replaced one addiction with another. And it chimed with my own experience. Battling exhaustion after my third child, and sitting opposite a fellow columnist who practically mainlined Coca-Cola, I fell into the habit of needing a Coke and chocolate bar before every deadline. Since I was filing copy almost every day, as a *Times* leader writer, my consumption of sugar was considerable. And pretty soon the chocolate bar was no longer a single small, elegant Green & Black's, but a string of Yorkie bars.

This kind of 'mindless eating' has been brought to life, hilariously and poignantly, in experiments by Brian Wansink of Cornell University. In one, he gave stale popcorn to two groups of cinemagoers.[39] One group got big buckets, the other got giant buckets so large that researchers assumed no one would finish them. When the movie ended, the people with giant buckets had scoured them clean – they'd consumed 50 per cent more popcorn than the others. When told this, most were astonished.

For decades, we were warned off saturated fat. A profitable industry grew up selling 'low-fat' processed foods. But these are a con. To make them tasty, manufacturers stuff them with carbohydrates and sugar. These create spikes in blood-sugar levels, which lead to cravings when blood sugar falls, along with the brain's chemical messenger, dopamine. Dopamine gives pleasure, but also regulates our self-control. So Big Food offering low-fat cakes is the equivalent of Big Tobacco offering low-tar cigarettes: they make us feel better about ourselves, while keeping us hooked.

I hope that doesn't sound hysterical. In 2015, there was a mortifying moment when I was called a 'health fascist' by one of the prime minister's other advisers. We had just come out of his office in Downing Street, where I had been arguing that we should tax sugary drinks. I was taken aback to hear myself described as fascist. But I believed we could no longer rely on exhortation to stem the obesity epidemic – we needed manufacturers to change their ingredients.

In 2016, the UK government announced that it would levy a tax on sugary drinks to tackle obesity. By the time the levy came into force two years later, most brands had already done what we had hoped they would: reformulate to avoid the tax, thus withdrawing substantial amounts of sugar from the supermarket shelves.[40] While a few customers have complained about taste – and Coca-Cola has refused to dilute its legendary Classic – many are switching to low-sugar products. This suggests that relatively small signals can change markets.

Reformulating food is much more complicated for the obvious reason that processed foods contain far more ingredients than drinks (if you remove all the sugar from a cake, it will simply collapse and look like a soufflé). But the UK government has already had some success in working with manufacturers to remove salt from processed foods. The same could be done for sugar — with the right combination of goodwill and political drive.

The assault on cigarettes was only partially about taxing and making them more expensive. It also involved health warnings on packets and restrictions on advertising. We need clear, unequivocal health warnings on processed food and drink in a universal language, not complex labels in small print that few of us can make sense of – especially when we're rushing down a supermarket aisle, vulnerable to pester power. One doctor recently told me that the government should be focusing on parents and grandparents, not child obesity. 'Unless the parents and grandparents lose weight,' she said, 'we've got no chance with the children.'

Parents and grandparents may not trust government, or the media, to tell them what to do. But they do trust doctors.

Persuading People to Lose Weight: In 20 Seconds

'Before you go,' says the GP, 'I just wanted to talk to you about your weight. You know the best way to lose weight is to go to a weight-watching programme[41] and that's available free on the NHS?'

Patient: 'Oh?'

Doctor: 'Yes, and I can refer you now if you are willing to give that a try?'

Patient: 'Yes, OK.'

Doctor: 'OK, what you need to do is take this envelope back outside, to the person who weighed you, and they will book you into the weight-loss course now.'

Patient: 'OK.'

Doctor: 'Good, but I'd like to see how you're getting on, so come and see me again in four weeks, please. OK?'

This simple conversation takes about 20 seconds – a tiny slice out of the doctor's appointment, held while you're putting on your coat and packing your bag. Yet it's rare. In England, almost nine in ten obese adults have never been offered any treatment.[42] Both British and American doctors report feeling too nervous to mention weight to obese patients. They don't know how to bring it up[43] – especially if they are overweight themselves. Yet our two nations top OECD league tables for obesity. The US is the fattest of 35 industrialised countries, just ahead of Mexico, and the UK lies in sixth place, ahead of any other country in Western Europe.

Given the clear health risks of obesity, you might think it would be a doctor's duty to raise the subject. But the prevailing view is that there's no point: that people either don't want to lose weight, or will just put it all back on again.

This isn't entirely correct. When a group of type 2 diabetics in Scotland were offered weight-loss programmes,[44] almost half ceased to be diabetic. They were completely cured and no longer need anti-diabetic drugs.

The 20-second conversation has proved similarly effective. When 137 primary care physicians in England were trained to use these exact phrases, an astonishing 83 per cent of patients agreed to participate in weight-loss schemes. A year later, the average person had lost a whopping 11kg.[45]

Only one in 500 patients complained that it was inappropriate for their doctor to raise the subject. Three-quarters said they hadn't even seriously considered losing weight before this conversation. But when help was offered by the trusted doctor – free, in a friendly, matter-of-fact way – they agreed. By investing a mere 20 seconds per patient (plus an hour and a half of online training), the doctors became the trusted gateway to an eight-week 'total diet replacement' programme, with personal support from specialists who don't drain time from medical staff. If that isn't a win–win, I don't know what is.

'We have overweight people coming to every medical facility,' says Susan Jebb, Professor of Diet and Population Health at the Nuffield Department of Primary Health Care Sciences, Oxford University. 'As body mass index has risen, so has the number of hospital appointments, GP appointments and prescriptions. We need to make every contact count.'

Jebb explains why weight-watching groups work. 'Everyone has already weighed themselves before they arrive,' she smiles. 'You can see them thinking how they're going to explain their weight loss or gain to the leader. The point is the external accountability. When people get structure, support and routine to help them lose weight, they can do brilliantly.'

Thirty years ago, doctors rarely asked about smoking, or offered patients help to give up. Now, they do so as a matter of routine. They need to start doing the same for obesity. All the more so because, like smoking, obesity hits the poor hardest.[46]

Unequal Ageing

'The rhetorical question is: how can you have two women, both aged 90, one of whom is physically fit and the other one is in a nursing home and can barely move?' Alan Walker, Professor of Social Policy and Social Gerontology at Sheffield University, has written. 'You can't explain those outcomes by genetics.

'There is nothing pre-determined about ageing, so there's no ageing gene, it's a matter of what biologists refer to as the environment, which is everything else. This means that we don't have to sit on the sidelines and just watch people age, we can give them advice about what a healthy outcome in later life will consist of, and how to ensure that if they do reach 100, their bodies and minds are in the best possible shape.'

Gerontologists like Walker are increasingly concerned about the inequalities which accumulate over a lifetime and are now exploding into view through the growing gaps in life expectancy and healthy life expectancy between older people. Not everyone has the money, knowledge or self-control to make the right lifestyle 'choices'. That's why, in my view, we need to curb the prevalence of junk food. We also need our health systems to focus on prevention.

Prevention Is Better Than Cure

There's something odd about the Geisinger health centre in Shamokin, Pennsylvania: it's also a food bank. In 2016, clinicians realised that many of their obese patients were below the poverty line and did not have enough access to fresh, nutritious food. So they decided to prescribe it.

The centre has a 'Fresh Food Farmacy', which dispenses enough fresh fruit, vegetables, whole grains and lean protein to feed overweight, diabetic patients and their families two healthy meals a day, for five days a week. They also provide recipes, and lessons on nutrition. One of those patients, Tom Shicowich, had to have his toe amputated, after his relentless diet of junk food and frozen meals became life-threatening. In the 18 months since he started the programme, Mr Shicowich has lost 60 pounds in weight and his blood-sugar levels have dropped below the danger zone.

Fresh Food Farmacy say they have lowered their patients' risk of serious diabetes complications by 40 per cent, and cut hospitalizations by 70 per cent. Their approach also saves money, by up to 80 per cent in some cases.[47]

Despite compelling evidence that diet and exercise can work miracles, far cheaper than drugs and with fewer side effects, Western healthcare systems spend far more on treating disease than preventing it. The NHS spends £97 billion a year on cure versus £8 billion on prevention; the ratio is similar in the US, the Netherlands and Norway, and even lower in Australia.[48] Modern health services were set up to treat disease, not to preserve health – and that's how they book the financial gains.

Public health is the Cinderella of government policy, the bit which gets cut when funding is tight. It's easy to quantify the costs of treating the sick, harder to judge the impact of public health interventions, whose pay-offs are often long term and don't improve the bottom line of any government department.

Healthy workers do, however, improve the bottom line of businesses, because absence rates fall and productivity rises. Employers will become increasingly interested in schemes run by insurers like Vitality, which offer rewards for healthy behaviours, and discounts on tracking devices like the Apple Watch, which can confirm how someone is living. Doctors can be powerful advocates for simple lifestyle changes – if they want to be. So can CEOs.

Younger Next Year?

Many of the limitations we experience as we get older are caused not by ageing itself, but by the way we live our lives – even from our thirties. Exercise is the equivalent of a miracle drug, which can reduce my risk of so many diseases, even dementia. The research is absolutely compelling: it jumps off the page. So why don't we all know about it?

Exercise is different from sport. As a child I was totally uncoordinated, was never in a team, and my parents' idea of exercise was leaving the car in a lay-by and strolling across a field to look at some ancient monument. Luckily, I did a degree in America, where aerobics was cool, and fell in love with it. I also had the good fortune to marry a fitness nut (our second date was in the gym). Now, I exercise to stay sane and to keep up with my three sons. But until now, I didn't realise what a good investment it has been.

We are held back from living better by our minds, by sedentary jobs and long commutes, by tempting junk foods and by doctors who, under pressure, find it easier to prescribe a pill than a change of life. Also, by the widespread myth in our societies that everything is downhill from 50. The Masters athletes, the Ikarians and the seventy-somethings still running in Illinois demonstrate that rapid physical decline is not inevitable. You won't banish wrinkles by joining a cycling club, but you will have more energy, exude more vitality, seem younger and in biological terms *be younger* if you eat right and lead a more active life.

The rich already know much of this – that's why many of them have personal trainers. A new term, MAMRI, or 'Middle-Aged Men Running Injured', has been coined to describe all the business executives who can be seen running madly – sometimes too madly – through big cities in pursuit of their youth.

Extra Time will be a Pyrrhic victory if we are doomed to spend years too weak to get out of a chair. Luckily, many of the keys to living longer better are within our control. We should be running exercise programmes for people of all ages to close the 'fitness gap'. We should tackle junk food as aggressively as we once tackled cigarettes. We should teach children about the revolutionary change in their life expectancy and what they can do to ensure a healthy and happy later life. But most of all, we need to stop confusing 'ageing' with loss of fitness. And be far more positive about what life can be.

4

No Desire to Retire

Don't give up the day job

'WHEN A CAR GETS old, everyone says you get a new one. But here, we work to keep the same cars running longer. We value the oldies,' chuckles Minuro Ishikawa, running his strong, tanned hands over a gleaming 1957 Toyota Crown, one of the vintage cars he restores for a living.

Aged 79, Ishikawa is a perfect exemplar of how to use Extra Time. He has outlived both the founder of Shinmei Automobile Co., who hired him, and the founder's son. He now works for the founder's grandson, Yasuhiro Kondo.

'He's irreplaceable,' says Kondo, a dark-haired, intense figure in his forties who treats Ishikawa rather like a favourite uncle. 'We are trying to train others to do these jobs, but they don't have his passion. This is the era of obsolescence, when younger people don't want to replace parts. Only he can conceptualise how to modify the parts.'

I'm in Toyota City, the car company's huge facility in central Japan. It contains ten factories, the Toyota stadium and Automobile Museum, and is home to around 400,000 people, many of whom depend on the car company for their livelihood. Ishikawa talks animatedly about how Shinmei's work boosts Toyota's reputation by taking in all brands of cars and rejuvenating them. He is what fashionable twenty-somethings would call an 'upcycler', fixing cars for which parts are no longer made by making bespoke parts from other materials. And he's in demand. He shows me his thick order book, which contains scribbled pictures of broken hoses and rusty chassis from dealerships all over the country.

Ishikawa doesn't look much like a garage mechanic. Dressed in pristine two-tone overalls, his silver hair neatly parted, he looks more like an ageing racing driver. He smiles a lot and keeps jumping up to bring me documents or to show me the modern, hybrid engine that he trains students on.

He is the first into the office every morning 'because,' he says firmly, 'the company is so important'. He adds that he is 'super-busy every day'.

As an 11-year-old boy, Ishikawa fell in love with machines. His mother used to sell sweet cakes from the back of a rickety old motorbike, which often broke down. On those occasions, she would ask Ishikawa to take it to the garage. At first, he would watch the men take it apart, clean it up and put it back together. 'Then I realised I could do it myself: I'd copy what I'd seen them do in the garage.' He didn't tell his mother. Later, he started buying up old taxicabs, fixing them and reselling them for a profit.

His passion is infectious. Most Saturdays, he takes part in volunteer workshops, getting schoolchildren to design go-karts. But 'what's most important,' he says as he drives me confidently to the train station in the fast lane, one hand lightly on the wheel and the other gesturing to emphasise his words, 'is teaching them how to greet people. Young kids today don't respond if you ask them questions. They need to learn how to listen. And,' he grins, 'how to clean up afterwards.'

Will he ever retire? 'No,' he says emphatically, 'not until I die.' Before he turned 60, the company president asked what he was planning to do in retirement.'I answered, "I'm not thinking of anything." He said, "In that case, why don't you keep coming here?" and that was that.'

His wife, he says, is delighted to have him out of the house. She makes him a packed lunch every day. 'I'm grateful,' he tells me. 'Grateful for my colleagues, for my work. Grateful to Toyota.'

Ishikawa feels especially lucky, because Japan has a retirement age of 60, which is usually mandatory, although some big companies offer staff an option to stay on another five years, on 40 per cent of their old salary.[1] Mandatory retirement is in some ways a logical response to Japan's traditional seniority system, where wages rise with age rather than merit, landing companies with a group of very expensive senior staff. It's almost impossible to fire anyone before 60, either from government or from a corporation, so retirement is a way for employers to extricate themselves from the seniority ratchet. But it's not ideal, in a country which is running out of workers.[2]

If the economic consequences are suboptimal, the social impact of the yawning gap between stopping work at 60 and living to 85 can be tragic. Executives who put in long hours as salarymen suddenly find themselves at home, bereft of office contacts, with resentful wives who call them 'gokiburi teishu' (cockroach husbands who do nothing). Some wives have developed ulcers from the stress of it, in what the Japanese psychiatrist Nobuo Kurokawa has called 'Retired Husband Syndrome'.[3] As a result, grey divorce is soaring.[4] In England and Wales divorce is declining in younger groups, but rising among the over-65s. Women, who are mostly the initiators,[5] are quailing at the prospect of looking at the same person for what could be 30 more years. While divorce can be empowering, it can also be impoverishing, and leads to more people living alone.

It might be better if so many people didn't feel like they'd hit a full stop.

What If Retirement Can Make You Old?

'When people retire at 60, they retreat,' says Fumio Takengi, Director of Silver Centre in Edogawa, east Tokyo, which helps older people find work. 'The common view in Japan has been that elderly people should passively receive welfare services. But this creates much unhappiness. The worst thing that can happen to a senior citizen is waiting to be helped. It does not build *ikigai* [reason for being].'

By providing part-time work, the Silver Centre movement restores purpose and connection to older citizens.

At the Edogawa Silver Centre, I find a group of wizened ladies, wearing flowery aprons they stitched themselves. Hands folded calmly in their laps, they sit expectantly round two big square tables. Racks of brown and white paper line one wall. It feels a bit like a kindergarten classroom.

'The work always changes,' says Mrs Shuize Ohata, 98, the oldest of the group. 'It keeps me a bright mind.' She has spent the morning tying gold elastic ribbons to be used in gift wrapping. It's a fiddly business, which saves the local factory time: their workers can just pop the ribbons over the presents. Piles of ribbons now lie neatly stowed in bundles, ready to be delivered.

Mrs Ohata has been coming here every week since her husband died, 20 years ago. She takes two buses to reach the centre and brings her own lunch: a bento box with salmon, eggs and rice balls. She says apologetically that she recently started buying the rice balls ready-made, rather than making them herself. Her face is soft and blotched with age, and she can barely see out of one eye, but she can still master the work, it seems. 'It's fun,' she says, clearly enjoying the attention bequeathed by her status as oldest senior. 'I get to chat with everybody.'

The manager pours a pile of brushes onto the table, which must be fitted onto sticks. Everyone leans forward as she demonstrates. 'I used to be a seamstress, so this suits me,' says Mrs Miyao, 88. She lives with her son and cooks for him, but he works long hours. 'I couldn't stay at home alone,' she says. 'Here, there's a different task every day. I like being useful.'

So, is this charity or is it work? As far as I can see, all the work is genuine. Silver Centres send members out to clean parks, pack goods in factories or to act as tour guides. The oldest member, a 101-year-old woman, looks after a historic building in Fukui. Companies genuinely value the help. In April and May, when corporate employees transfer to new jobs, older people with good calligraphy skills are in demand to draw the official handmade certificates of congratulations. It's a time-consuming process, which requires grinding the inkstone and perfecting each brushstroke.

The first Silver Centre was founded in 1975 by a Tokyo University professor and some retired friends who wanted to supplement their income, maintain their health and contribute to society. They encountered enormous resistance from the authorities, who feared older workers would displace younger ones. Today, the government subsidises Silver Centres, but it will still not let them provide full-time jobs. There are no formal employment contracts: the workers are 'members' of the Centre and are paid 'dividends', not 'wages'.

This approach seems a little quaint, given that Japan's productivity will eventually suffer unless it makes more use of older workers. But the Silver Centres have a broader goal. 'It's not just doing a job and getting paid,' says Mr Takengi, 'it's building camaraderie and helping others. Local people see someone cleaning the park devotedly, they stop and talk to them. Their effort is appreciated by the local community and leads to *ikigai*. Your salary isn't everything: having a place to shine matters.'

This place is clearly a lifeline. A bus ride away from Funibori station in east Tokyo, the Centre is housed in a run-down side street. Yet Mr Takengi tells me that an astounding 2,400 people come here every month, to report on how they've been doing, work-wise and physically. 'Ninety-three per cent of our members are very healthy,' he says. 'We believe that our system helps keep them that way.' And perhaps it does. For research increasingly shows that purpose and social connection are good for us. We may need to change the type of job we do as we grow older, but most of us will need to keep going – and earning.

The Mid-Life Start-Ups

Entrepreneurs are coming to the rescue. In 2017, entrepreneurs over 50 employed more people in UK start-ups than the under-50s.[6] In the US, 55- to 65-year-olds are 65 per cent more likely to start a business than 20- to 34-year-olds.[7]

These are not all hobbies, or fake consultancies to tote a business card. According to the *Harvard Business Review* (*HBR*), older entrepreneurs actually have a much higher success rate than younger ones. The average age of founders of the highest-growth start-ups in the US is now 45, which rises to 47 if you remove social media but keep biotech.[8] 'If you were faced with two entrepreneurs and knew nothing about them besides their age, you would do better, on average, betting on the older one,' the HBR writes.

Youth can be an elixir of brilliance. Bill Gates, Steve Jobs, Jeff Bezos, Sergey Brin and Larry Page all founded their businesses very young and made history. But there may be something to be said for maturity too. Jobs was 52 by the time that Apple introduced the iPhone, its most profitable gadget. Bezos was 45 when Amazon's future market capitalisation growth rate hit its peak.

Not everyone has woken up to these new kids on the block. Paul Graham, who cofounded Y Combinator, has talked about 'the cut-off in investors' heads' being '32'. Venture capitalists who reject the oldies are missing out.

This later life dynamism comes in the nick of time. Jobs for life have gone. It was in the 1970s that pensions morphed from being seen as a support for dignity in old age into more of a reward for loyal employees, gracefully making way for a younger generation.

Early retirement became entrenched, even as life expectancy was rising.

Today, the numbers no longer stack up. Longevity has sent many pension schemes into deficit. New York City now has more retired policemen than working ones, and spends more on ex-cops' pensions than current cops' wages.[9] In 2017, a report forecast that New York City's annual pension contributions would soon displace social services as the second-largest spending category in the city budget.[10]

Private pension schemes have shifted from defined-benefit plans, where workers get a fixed income in retirement to defined-contribution plans, where future returns are far less secure and workers shoulder the risk. Not knowing when the end will come, some react by spending less than they could, depriving the economy of their money. Others find themselves with smaller pensions than they expected.[11]

It's a recipe for anxiety.

Governments have moved gingerly to raise pension ages, afraid to upset the burgeoning grey vote but also conscious of their obligations to citizens who were, arguably, mis-sold an expectation of a different world. After the financial crisis, 18 OECD countries raised the retirement age.[12] But the rate of those rises is not keeping pace with projected increases in life expectancy.

The obvious answer is for more of us to work longer. Intriguing differences between countries suggest that this is perfectly possible. In New Zealand, 78 per cent of 55- to 64-year-olds are currently in work. That figure is 76 per cent in Sweden and 84 per cent in Iceland.[13] Yet it's only 64 per cent in the UK and Australia, and 62 per cent in the US.[14] There's no great difference between the jobs available in those countries: the UK is currently enjoying historically low rates of unemployment. Nor is there any fundamental difference in the abilities or health of their populations. If the UK matched the employment rate of New Zealand, it could add almost 9 per cent to annual GDP.[15] (It's worth noting that New Zealand and the Nordic countries have put a lot of weight on flexible working, and digital skills training – two things which older people say they need.)

Longevity economists Andrew Mason and Ronald Lee have calculated that if people in the 'older countries', like Germany, Japan and Spain, were to delay retirement by 2.5 years per decade between 2010 and 2050, that would be sufficient to offset the economic effects of demographic changes.[16]

With physically demanding occupations in decline, it's reasonable to assume that people who are physically able could work longer – if they can find a job.

The New Trend: 'Unretirement'

'I was terrified,' says Laura Dobbs, who retired from her full-time job as a marketing executive in Pennsylvania at the age of 70. 'I knew I had to step down sooner or later, it was punishing work, but the job was a big part of who I was. My biggest fear was not being relevant. I thought, I'm finally going to be shelved someplace, I'm going to lose my identity.' Now 75, Dobbs has recently started a part-time job closer to home: 'I just wasn't ready to give up,' she says. 'It's good to be needed.'

Dobbs is part of a quiet movement of older Anglo-Saxons who are trooping back to work. One in four Americans and Brits now 'unretire' after having officially retired.[17] Their reasons are both financial (men with mortgage debt make up a significant segment) and psychological: a desire for routine and camaraderie. One survey found a significant number of people saying they had gone back to work after they'd been asked to 'lend a hand'. Australia's rate of 'unretirement' is lower, at around 10 per cent.[18]

The 'unretired' tend to be highly educated. The more qualified you are, the more likely you are to find a job – and the more likely you are to want one, it seems. RAND's American Working Conditions survey[19] found that 60 per cent of retired college graduates would be interested in working again if they found the right job, compared with only 40 per cent without a college degree. This isn't surprising. Inspiring literature about 'finding yourself' in your second phase may resonate less if you have bad knees, hostile colleagues, and your only option is to keep working the checkout.

Studies broadly suggest that if you enjoy your job, and will miss the contact it brings, your health may suffer after you retire. That applies to many professionals, whose jobs are hugely bound up with identity and self-esteem. The most vibrant people I've met over 60, who seem to be getting the most from their Extra Time, are still working. They're not necessarily doing the same job as they were at 50, though.

This is not true in all cases, especially if you're in a low-paid job which is repetitive and stressful. Experts suggest that people who hate their job can benefit from giving up – especially if they use the Extra Time to improve their physical fitness. But even those people are advised not to give up for ever. RAND economist Dr Nicole Maestas has tracked people who leave jobs with a lot of stress and physical demands, whose 'interactions with people at work are strained or hostile'. They go through a cycle of burnout and recovery, after which time, she suggests, they could be ready to start again.[20]

The problem, though, is how to rejoin the rat race. As one expert told me: 'If you want to stay in work, don't retire. It's far harder to get back in.'

The Hidden Jobless

David Wilson, 58, hasn't worked for the past two years. He was made redundant from the Civil Service and replaced by someone younger. 'The longer I'm out, the harder it is to get back in,' he says. 'Each job I try for, I'm getting the same response: "we have other qualified candidates with more recent experience". I'm close to giving up.'

This story chimes with research suggesting that some employers would rather hire someone with no relevant experience than someone who has been unemployed for more than a year. It's the same story in Michigan, where Mike Yack, 62, can't find another job since being laid off by General Motors.[21] 'I am physically able,' he told Reuters. 'I'd be open to anything – learning a new trade or something. But,' he continued, 'the opportunity is not there. I don't expect top wages, but I am not going to work for 10 dollars an hour.'

If David Wilson and Mike Yack give up looking, they won't show up in unemployment figures. This raises an important question: how many officially retired people are unhappily retired?

A Reuters/Ipsos poll in 2014[22] found an astounding 40 per cent of Americans who described themselves as 'retired' saying they would have preferred to keep working. Thirty per cent said they would go back to work if the right job came along, but 34 per cent *had given up looking*.

Opportunity is clearly affected by where you live, but also by prejudice. In survey after survey, older workers are thought to be variously, both slow and 'overqualified'; likely to take more time off sick (in fact, the opposite is true) and resistant to training (hard to test, since older workers are rarely offered any). Older people are more loyal than footloose youngsters, but even that can be turned into a negative image: of plodders with nowhere else to go.

When researchers at the UK's Anglia Ruskin University applied for jobs using fake CVs, they found that an older worker was four times less likely to be called for interview than a 28-year-old with ostensibly identical skills.[23] A similar exercise in America[24] received 35 per cent fewer responses to CVs sent in by the fake applicants aged 64–66, and 19 per cent fewer responses to those pretending to be 49–51, than those aged 29 to 31.

In 2018, a UK parliamentary committee concluded that the talents of more than a million people over 50 are being wasted, because of bias and outdated hiring practices.[25] The committee heard evidence of firms advertising for 'energy', 'enthusiasm' or 'dynamism', then sifting out older people's CVs. 'They are not thinking, "We do not want an older person,"' a representative of the charity Age UK explained. 'They are just thinking, "We want someone who is x, y and z." Then they apply those characteristics and come up with someone who is probably not an older person.'

Sometimes it's more blatant. A California jury heard the case of fire chief George Corley, sacked aged 58 after an unblemished 38 years and replaced by a much younger, less experienced division chief.[26] The court heard that the San Bernadino Country Fire Service had used a ploy known as 'freeway therapy' – posting people to far-flung places with long commutes – to get them to retire. The jury rightly found in favour of Mr Corley – and he found work in another district.

Conscious or unconscious, if we don't do something about these prejudices, we will limit the productive capacity of our economy.

Why bother about old people, you may ask, in the face of automation? With big-tech scything through industries, swapping us for algorithms, shouldn't we put youngsters first?

The belief that older people keep young ones out of a job is hugely influential. But it's what economists rather rudely call the 'lump of labour fallacy', because there isn't a fixed number of jobs in the economy, and older and younger workers are not readily substituted for each other. Men didn't lose jobs when women surged into the workforce after the Second World War. Instead, the economy grew. Countries where many older workers are employed generally have high employment rates for younger workers too – and vice versa.[27] In the US and China, one study found no evidence that employing older people altered job opportunities or wage rates for younger workers over a 40-year period.[28]

Here's the paradox: just as we enter the Fourth Industrial Revolution, when AI, big data and robotics are about to transform the way we live, demography is creating skill shortages. In the UK, a third of qualified nurses are set to retire in the next ten years[29] and half of farm holders are over 50.[30]

Robots may indeed threaten our jobs. But as populations age, employers will be fighting to find enough humans.

The Robots May Be Coming, But We Are Running Out of Humans

In 2007, the management team at BMW's biggest European car-making plant, Dingolfing in Germany, were worried. Dingolfing is where the 3, 4, 5, 6 and 7 BMW Series cars roll off the assembly line. It also makes car bodies for Rolls-Royce. These are top-quality products made with high-precision engineering.

Nikolaus Bauer, head of the power train plant at Dingolfing, and his production managers, could see that their workforce was getting older. With the German Chamber of Commerce predicting that Germany would soon lack 400,000 skilled workers in manufacturing,[31] they knew the pool of talent was shrinking.

Assembling cars and components is physically challenging and highly skilled. Bauer and his managers didn't want to lose their skilled older workers just because they weren't as strong or flexible as they used to be. And as the biggest employer in Lower Bavaria, they also felt a responsibility to the community. So they began an experiment which was to disprove almost every assumption about older workers.

Bauer and his managers chose one of the production lines, which produced rear-axle gearboxes, and turned it into an 'older' line. They changed the team members on that line, so that almost half were over 50 and the average age was 47. Next, they held workshops, where they quizzed the men about their aches and pains, and asked what they would change to make life easier. One of the earliest suggestions was to put in wood flooring, which reduced exposure to jolts from static electricity. They added revolving barbershop chairs to ease strain and magnifying lenses to counteract failing eyesight. The team ended up making 70 changes to improve productivity, including more rapid job rotation to reduce physical strain.

Initially, the project was unpopular, including with the older workers. It was derided as 'the pensioners' line' – until managers publicly joined in with the team's daily stretching exercises on the shop floor. It didn't take long for those exercises to spread to the rest of the factory – or for the cynics to shut up. For the results were extraordinary.[32]

The new, older team worked faster than the one it replaced. Productivity went up by 7 per cent. Absenteeism dropped from 7 per cent to 2 per cent, below the factory average. And the number of assembly defects fell to zero. This was far beyond what anyone had expected – including the workers themselves. And it didn't even cost that much: about 40,000 euros. The cost of hiring and training new staff, instead of keeping the old ones, would have been significantly more.

The BMW experiment is partly a story about how technological advances will revolutionise our ability to do hard, physical jobs. Ford is now testing lightweight exoskeleton vests in some of its US plants, which help toiling workers of all ages to lift things more easily and avoid shoulder injury. But the BMW story is also about belonging. The BMW workers essentially built their own line. Many reported having more energy, and I don't think it was just because their knees weren't aching any more. They started turning up, without fail. They worked faster. And this might have had something to do with the fact that they felt needed, felt they were a vital part of the company's future, not a bunch of guys on their way out.

Spare a Thought for the CEOs

'I've always been against automated chronological dates to farm people out,' Lee Iacocca, the legendary auto exec who ran Chrysler, told *Wired* magazine. 'The union would always say, "Make room for the new blood, there aren't enough jobs to go around." Well, that's a hell of a policy to have. I had people at Chrysler who were 40 but acted 80, and I had 80-year-olds who could do everything a 40-year-old can. Age gives experience. Besides, it takes you until about 50 to know what the hell is going on in the world.'

Age has always been a lousy predictor of performance. Anyone who's ever managed people has encountered a version of Mr Iacocca's Mr X, who is '40 but acts 80'. Some of us – ahem – may even have passed Mr X on to another department, by writing him an undeservedly good reference. His lacklustre performance should have been sorted out long before. But few of us enjoy confrontation.

Well-meaning campaigners for the rights of older workers sometimes make it sound as if everyone over 60 is a tremendously valuable resource. But that hurts the cause, because it's simply not true. Clare, a sprightly 70-year-old who was viewed with suspicion by younger colleagues when she joined a new enterprise, told me this: 'They'd only just got rid of someone called Sue, who was 60 and hopeless. They were afraid I was another Sue. Who can blame them?'

For managers, retirement has often been a convenient way out when there are performance issues (Sue might have improved, had anyone bothered to challenge her, instead of giving her a lukewarm annual performance appraisal). It has also been a way to cap costs. Employers face a genuine conundrum when someone senior has grown stale in a role, but expects their pay to keep rising. Even with flatter hierarchies, we still harbour deep-seated expectations that older people will be more senior and better paid. But if we all want to work longer, it's simply inconceivable that our pay can keep going up. If it does, we will price ourselves out of the workforce.

Let's face it, when the word 'dynamic' appears in adverts it is code not just for 'young', but also for 'cheap'. That may not be fair, but it is a reality we need to appreciate if we are to genuinely help older people.

For all its drawbacks, Japan's mandatory retirement age does make it normal for older people to take a pay cut. It's a blunt instrument and not one I'm advocating. But in the US and Europe, age discrimination laws can make it feel risky to have an open conversation about whether someone would move sideways, or accept a lower wage. Until there is a safe space to discuss these issues, too many people may be moved on simply for getting old. In the US, where employers pay for health insurance, older workers can cost five times as much to insure as younger ones.[33] Professor Laura Carstensen, Director of the Stanford Longevity Center, describes a meeting she called with company bosses to discuss how they could get more out of older workers. To her horror, most of the executives round the table wanted to know how to manage graceful exits.

Employment is a two-way street. I can't think of anything less likely to endear older people to employers than the insistence of the UK parliamentary committee I referred to earlier, that everyone over 50 must be offered flexible working as soon as they're hired. Some companies may well choose to attract people with such offers, especially to staff looking after elderly parents. But to insist on special dispensation for everyone in their fifties simply reinforces the view that fifty-something people are different, and more demanding, when we ought to be fighting to show that they are the same, and just as good. Many millennials want flexible work too: why single out the over-50s who may, in fact, be gunning for a full-time role after the kids have grown up?

There is a danger in thinking backwards from retirement. If you assume you'll retire at 60, you may start to mentally disengage at 55. And your employer may do likewise. Alicia Munnell, Director of the Center for Retirement Research at Boston College, has given this advice to over-50s worried about their future: 'Stay with your current employer, don't hurl yourself onto the job market. Tell your employer you're committed for the long term, and you'd like to get training.' She's also firm about part-timers: 'If you portray yourself as a short-timer, your job gets less interesting. You almost define your job away.' A neat riposte to the current orthodoxy about flexibility.

For some CEOs, thinking about how to motivate older workers is simply part of being human.

Looking Like Your Customers

In the fast-moving City of London, home to some of the world's biggest banks and insurance companies, grey hair is usually a sign that you're on the way out – or you're on the board. But Andy Briggs, the tall, rangy CEO of Aviva UK Insurance, actively wants more grey hair in his business.

It's a Friday afternoon in March 2018, and the City is bristling with talk of the gender pay gap. Three years ago, the British government demanded that companies report on pay differences between their male and female staff.[34] Now, there are only two weeks to go to the deadline. Some of the banks around here – we're in the heart of the financial district and I can see the iconic Gherkin building out of the window – are nervous about how their numbers will be received.

But that's not what is energising Mr Briggs. Aviva UK has already revealed its gender pay gap, and it's better than most financial service companies. This CEO is concerned about a different kind of gap: not between men and women, but between young and old.

Andy Briggs has pledged to increase the number of over-50s that Aviva UK employs by 12 per cent and to publish data about the age of his workforce to measure progress. If he succeeds, a quarter of Aviva UK's 16,000 staff will be over 50 by 2022.

Why? Like BMW, Aviva sees a looming skills deficit: '1.5 million people leave the workforce each year in the UK, and only 750,000 enter,' says Briggs, stretching out his legs under the coffee table. 'Immigration has been filling much of the gap, before Brexit, but Brexit brings this into focus.' He is also acutely aware of the hardship that some pensioners may face: 'As a pension company, we see the need for people to work longer and save more.'

But it's not just about numbers. Briggs believes that 'more diverse workforces make better decisions'. And, he says, older people are more loyal: 'A 50-year-old man is four times less likely to leave in the next five years than a twenty-something.'

Briggs tells me the story of Ken, a former civil servant who joined Aviva at the age of 56, to work in its life insurance claims team. 'It's typically 60-year-olds who ring up that team,' he explains, 'about a loved one who's died, or about their own critical illness. It's difficult.' Most of the Aviva staff were much younger than the customers. 'Ken picked up digital skills from our youngsters,' he says, 'but he also helped them understand the callers. The department is all the better for it.'

With one in five over-50s now caring for an elderly relative,[35] the company now offers carers generous paid and unpaid leave. 'You wouldn't hear a business saying to a pregnant woman, you can have the day off to have the baby, but you need to be at work the day before and the day after,' says Briggs, emphatically. 'This is the same.'

The company looked at what else it could do to attract older applicants. 'We looked at our adverts,' says Briggs, 'and everyone was young, fit and smiling. We didn't want people over 50 to think "it's not for me".' So Aviva's adverts now include older people – and they are smiling too.

Rewriting the Career Timetable in Our Heads

When I started researching this book, I was amazed to find that almost every piece of data about 'older' workers started at age 50. This makes 50 feel like the last staging post before the cliff edge. Yet by the time we reach 50, some of us will be only halfway through our lives. And nowhere near the end of our careers.

If we are to make full use of Extra Time, we are going to have to rewrite the career timetable. It's still a pretty universal assumption that we'll work flat out in our thirties, 'make it' in our forties and peak in our fifties. Yet this is crazy. First, because few of us will want to plateau in our fifties, with so much left to give. Second, because it squashes the time of greatest intensity in our careers into the period marked 'child-rearing'.

For parents, somewhere between the late twenties and early forties lies a period of sleepless nights and school runs, followed by teenage angst. But these are also the most pressured years of our working lives. The peak earning age for graduates in the US and UK is 48 for men, and 39 for women.[36] If you haven't scaled the ladder by then, it can feel like you're not going to.

To make matters worse, many big firms still identify their rising stars around the age of 30. It's at that point that you get on the partner track, or you start to receive leadership training. The stakes are high. Many ambitious people have their feet clamped so hard on the career accelerator that they have too little time for their families in their thirties, only to get spat out at 60 when they've still got plenty of energy and their children don't need them any more.

This system leaves almost everyone in a state of regret about what they didn't do. And it's woefully inefficient. The traditional career timetable dramatically shrinks the talent pool, by excluding anyone who doesn't stick to it. It's especially unfair to women, who still tend to shoulder the bulk of caring responsibilities. And it makes no sense when people are living longer and in better health.

I know so many able women who are fed up with the idea that the only real progress has to be perpetual upward motion. There's a time for that, but it should be in our own time. Personally, I have been tremendously lucky. After my first child was born, I left my corporate job and became a journalist. For the next 14 years, I worked four days a week, and was able to build a new career around motherhood, with wonderfully supportive bosses. I didn't take another full-time job until my third son was six.

Along the way, I became acutely aware that to fulfil my role as a mother, I had to sidestep promotions. With a husband working all hours and travelling a lot, I felt that something would break if I took on more responsibilities. The world of newspapers was pretty forgiving. But I know so many women in professional jobs who have found themselves written out of the script permanently, because they were reluctant to take promotion while their children were small. For many, the killer was international travel. You can hold a household together working five days a week but if you are frequently abroad, things fall apart.

The wasted talent at the school gates is tragic. A few visionary law firms and banks are now pioneering 'returner' schemes to support and entice professional women back to work after long absences. PwC, the accounting firm, has estimated that this could add £1.7 billion to the British economy.[37] But such schemes are few and far between. And there is no equivalent for women with fewer qualifications, although they are the ones who could benefit most.

If 50 is the cliff edge, what about giving people a Mid-Career MOT, to help them take stock of where they are in their lives?[38] We get careers advice at 16, when we haven't got a clue, so why not advise people who have already experienced the workplace and know what they're good at? A Mid-Career MOT could be a positive way to think about Extra Time: assess skills, health and finances, while emphasising the fact that most 50-year-olds are still mid-career, not slowing down.

Japan's Silver Centres already provide some of this. They don't just find people jobs, they also act as brokers, developing profiles of each client's skills and experience and matching them to vacancies. Which surely proves that it's never too late to get careers support.

Welcome to the Multi-Generational Workforce

On 8 February 1996, John Perry Barlow – Grateful Dead songwriter, cattle-rancher and internet campaigner – was attending the World Economic Forum in Davos, Switzerland. A less likely fit with the world's business elite would be hard to find. Barlow was a craggy-faced hippie who dressed in black, had dropped acid with Timothy Leary and co-founded the Electronic Frontier Foundation, the powerful digital rights group which argued for internet freedoms. He was also a brilliant wordsmith and a visionary. And what he wrote that day, from his hotel room in the Alps, electrified the world. It was a letter to the American government, entitled 'A Declaration of the Independence of Cyberspace'.

'Governments of the Industrial World, you weary giants of flesh and steel, I come from Cyberspace, the new home of Mind,'[39] he wrote. 'On behalf of the future, I ask you the past to leave us alone. You are not welcome among us. You have no sovereignty where we gather.'

Barlow's arguments for cyberspace liberty were powerful, as was this sentence in his Declaration: 'You are terrified of your own children, since they are natives in a world in which you will always be immigrants.'

That sentence drew an enduring line between the generations. Between digital natives, who grew up in the digital age, and digital immigrants, who only became familiar with technology as adults. It's a powerful concept, which speaks to an important truth. But it has also become a destructive prejudice, used to dismiss the 'immigrants' as people who will never be savvy enough, never quite get it, always be behind. Solely because they are older.

Employers I meet often confide their worry that the old won't 'get' social media. Older people themselves fear that they lack tech insight which they can never acquire, because they're not 'natives'. Some are so afraid, it puts them off trying. Tech speak can be a bar to entry as effective as any degree qualification, and as insidious as racism.

'They had a much greater understanding of technology than I did,' admits one 72-year-old business executive, who offered her considerable skills to a non-profit enterprise where the average age was 29. 'They were generous in helping me to use things like Skype, which I hadn't used before. They'd say things like "you picked that up pretty well, much better than we expected". It was a bit patronising, to be honest. I felt that these bright young people thought I was fine, but that they had more relevant experience than me. But they knew nothing about management, and I did.'

She also felt there was a gulf in vocabulary. 'Millennials will put "ality" on the end of words,' she says, bemused. 'They say things like functionality instead of function. We kept saying to each other, "I don't understand what you mean".' As a result, she feels, they weren't sure how to deal with her: 'They were hesitant to disagree with me – but I'd have much preferred it if they had.' Eventually, she took her skills elsewhere.

These differences need not be terminal. But unless they are aired, it will be harder to get more generations working under one roof.

There is a growing buzz about the benefits of an 'age diverse workforce'.[40] Haig Nalbantian, an economist with the consultancy Mercer, has found that older workers are slower at some tasks but often more emotionally stable than their younger counterparts, and better at handling tense situations. When old and young work together, errors decrease and productivity rises. Similar findings by Axel Börsch-Supan, of Germany's Max-Planck Institute, suggest that productivity can actually increase with age, when it comes to interacting with customers.[41] CVS Health, the US drug store chain, is actively hiring staff between 55 and 99 to match its shoppers.[42]

It's not all plain sailing. Researchers found that a widening disparity in age can lead to resentment,[43] if an older person gets what is thought of as a 'young job' – in IT or sales, for example – or a youngster is promoted rapidly into an 'old job' – in senior management or finance. There may be mutters of 'Hmm ... will he be able to keep up?' or 'Hmm ... isn't she a bit young for that?'[44] For CEOs, it's a minefield.

The New Gigs

'This is freedom and it keeps me young,' says Ken Barillas, 64, in whose Lincoln Town car I'm Uber-pooling through San Francisco. The money isn't as steady as in his old job in logistics, but he likes being in control of his time. Mr Barillas is saving up for a new boat – his hobby is fishing. But even when he's made enough, he thinks he'll keep working – at least until Uber switches to self-driving cars. 'It's the conversation I love,' he smiles. 'A robot won't tell you what I just did about Princess Diana!'

The twenty-first century may increasingly come to resemble the early twentieth century, when most workers were freelancers, working for multiple customers. A third of Brits over pension age are self-employed.[45] A quarter of all Uber drivers in the US are over 50.[46] In the UK, the wonderfully named start-up No Desire to Retire finds freelance work for the over-50s. In the US, insurance professionals in their sixties and seventies are working for Work At Home Vintage Employees, created by 64-year-old Sharon Emek. Others are finding work through Retired Brains, founded by 76-year-old Art Koff.

But whether the gig economy of independent contractors represents exploitation or liberation depends on your bargaining power. A student who came to one of my Harvard study groups said something which has stayed with me. 'At my father's engineering firm,' he said, 'lots of senior guys retire and come back as consultants. But Ellie on the front desk, she didn't get to come back. Nor did Barbara, the secretary. Why don't they get the same chances?'

In Extra Time, professional people can 'unretire', prosper as entrepreneurs and command premiums. Those with fewer skills are more likely to retire early and less likely to have saved enough for retirement. Even if they're not replaced by technology, they don't have the networks to find another job. The prospects of those with fewer skills are looking increasingly bleak, *at every age*. That's the real divide: not between young and old but skilled and networked, and unskilled without networks.

In this new world more and more of us will be like actors, auditioning for different roles in insecure lives. Maybe we will need what actors have: agents who help us pitch and protect our rights. Or start-up trade unions which understand people who have several jobs, not one, and can provide the kind of networks which disappeared with working men's clubs.

We may also need places to work, with companionship and office facilities. Older workers are joining the surge into co-working spaces – like Second Home in London, StationW in Paris and Camaraderie Coworking in Toronto. Rohan Silva, founder of Second Home, saw a 40 per cent increase in applications from people over 60 in 2017. 'We've been blown away by the numbers,' he says. 'This group clearly has no intention of slowing down, and wants to use our spaces and community to help them start new businesses.'

Is It Fair to Ask Everyone to Work Longer?

Given that we are living longer, it seems reasonable to ask people to work longer, to maintain the same share of life spent in retirement as previous generations. But what if people are not living longer equally?

In rich countries, the wealthiest and most educated workers can expect to live around a decade longer than the poorest, and in better health. If we ask them all to work longer, some will end up with much less time in retirement.

Some fascinating research under way in the US,[47] by the National Academies of Sciences Committee on the Long Run Macroeconomic Effects of the Aging US Population, looks at how the growing gap in life expectancy could affect lifetime benefits from federal welfare programmes. The authors calculate that the top 20 per cent of earners born in 1960 stand to earn a stunning $130,000 more in lifetime benefits, net of tax, than the bottom 20 per cent. Even though the top earners will pay more in tax over their lives, they will accrue more social security benefits simply by living so much longer. Lower-income people are eligible for extra disability benefits, but these won't be enough to stop the benefits system becoming less generous to them.

Until now, governments have raised retirement ages on the basis of *mean* life expectancy (adding up everyone's life expectancies and dividing by the population). They have not formally considered the big potential mortality differences between different groups. But if pension ages keep rising, we must also find ways to protect the poorest. The National Academies of Sciences Committee found that the only policy which could restore the balance between the richest and poorest would be to reduce social security benefits for the top half of all earners. That would be a drastic change to what has, until now, been a universal benefit. But that's the kind of change we must consider.

One radical idea which has become very fashionable is universal basic income (UBI): a flat payment to everyone which would be enough to live on, which would end the complex patchwork of welfare benefits. Exponents argue this would reduce inequalities and provide a secure platform to smooth difficult transitions in life. While superficially attractive, UBI would be extremely expensive –

which is why Finland recently dropped it, after a pilot.[48] But I have another problem with it. The more I think about it, the more I find the idea of telling people 'don't worry, we'll pay you not to work' is anathema. I would rather try to keep people in work, which has so many benefits for mental wellbeing – not accelerate the flow out of it. But if we're going to do that, we have to radically redesign education.

In the Fourth Industrial Revolution We Will Need a Fourth Stage of Education

When I invited the deputy prime minister of Singapore to lunch, I hadn't expected to end up talking about flower arranging.

Tharman Shanmugaratnam is a clever, articulate politician who has held many ministerial positions in Singapore and has always kept a close eye on social mobility: 'as Singaporeans, our whole identity rests on the fact that everyone has a fair chance to move up'. In 2014, he launched the SkillsFuture programme, the most ambitious learning initiative in the world, to address the twin challenges of ageing and the jobs revolution.

Singapore did not need to redesign its education system. Its schools are the envy of the world, consistently coming top, or near the top, of international league tables.[49] Yet the nation is ageing dramatically. Right now, one in eight Singaporeans is over 65. In only 15 years' time, that will be one in four.[50] Tharman's solution is to create a true meritocracy of continuous learning, where your future isn't limited by the grades you got as a teenager. Under SkillsFuture, every citizen over the age of 25 gets a S$500 (around £320) credit to pay for approved courses. That credit will never expire, and will be topped up at intervals by the government. There are extra subsidies for people over 40, and discounts for employers who sponsor workers to take courses in everything from fashion to blockchain.

Around the table there was a sharp intake of breath as we all realised how much this must cost. The idea of a government writing a lifetime cheque, which could accumulate and be cashed in even by centenarians, was amazing. 'Surely you don't want to pay 90-year-olds to do flower arranging?' one of my team ventured, choosing the most frivolous subject he could think of. Tharman smiled. 'If it keeps people occupied and their minds alert, we should consider it,' he said earnestly. 'The absolute returns on investment matter less than changing the national mindset.' Of course he is right: the widow learning to arrange flowers in a convivial setting will be happier, and probably end up costing the state less, than one who stares out of a lonely window.

Tharman's insight is that learning should be a continuous process which binds all the age groups together, not just a silo for young or old. It's never too early to start – his government is also heavily subsidising weaker learners in pre-school – nor is it ever too late to stop.

'RIP the three-stage working life,' wrote Andrew Scott and Lynda Gratton in their excellent book *The 100-Year Life*. The old model of 'education – work – leisure' no longer fits, the authors argued, when people are living so much longer. All countries need their own version of SkillsFuture: one in which age is irrelevant, and what matters is interest and aptitude.

EQ Will Be as Important as IQ

In 1995, the *New York Times* writer Daniel Goleman popularised the idea of 'emotional intelligence' in his book of the same name. He described the importance of empathy, listening and motivation for careers and relationships, and argued that 'EQ' (which stands for emotional quotient) is as important a factor in success as IQ.

As AI and big data start to take over many cognitive tasks, Goleman's message seems more important than ever. We already know that AI can diagnose and predict some diseases better than doctors, for example. Doctors won't disappear, but we will increasingly prize their bedside manner, empathy and their ability to explain the complexities of probability as genetic tests go mainstream. We will value their EQ, as well as their IQ.

One job where EQ is already paramount, or should be, is caring. The demand for carers will increase sharply as populations age, and the skills most needed will be the ones that, I will argue in Chapter 8, robots cannot provide: emotional resilience, intuition and empathy. Yet people who do caring jobs are often looked down on, or described as 'unskilled', because they have talents which are not 'academic'.

I saw this for myself when I travelled around England in 2013, interviewing junior nurses and care workers for an independent review I was commissioned to carry out by the Department of Health.[51] I met hundreds of these wonderful staff, working in hospitals or helping care for people at home, and was struck by the extraordinary maturity and resilience that is needed to walk into the home of an elderly stranger, establish a relationship and help them take a shower. I was surprised and upset by the patronising attitudes that some senior nurses and doctors had to the junior healthcare assistants in hospitals who were 'only' making tea, lifting patients out of bed or helping them eat. Yet these are the people who spend most time at the bedside, who are most likely to notice when something is wrong and can make all the difference to whether a patient feels secure or afraid.

The good hospitals wanted to promote their best junior staff, having watched them in action on the wards. But the ladder had been knocked away by the demand that all registered nurses should have university degrees. Our traditional university system leaves little flexibility for women (they were mostly middle-aged women) who didn't do well at school.[52] They might have successfully brought up children, managed households and cared for their own ageing parents, but they are not thought 'academic' enough to be promoted – even though they have the compassion that patients are crying out for.

Developing EQ will require very different kinds of education to memorising facts and honing cognitive skills. It will not happen through traditional universities, which have a vested interest in restricting entry, because their currency is prestige. Andy Haldane, Chief Economist at the Bank of England, has suggested we need a 'multiversity': an institution with multiple entry points at all ages, which teaches technical and emotional skills, not only conventional 'cognitive' ones. This is an idea which seems right for our times. The 'multiversity' could offer a second chance to people whose grades were not great at school. It could provide filmed lectures, online quizzes and user chats through MOOCs (massive open online courses). But most importantly, it would build on what we can do, not remind us of what we can't.

The Age of No Retirement

For many of us, retirement at 60, 65 or earlier will become an outmoded concept. It needs to, if our economies are to prosper and if we ourselves are to remain involved and productive. It will also be in the interests of companies to retain good staff for longer – who will increasingly look like their customers. CEOs could start by challenging their own notion of the career timetable; offering staff mid-career MOTs and embracing talented mothers (and hands-on fathers) who want to return.

That does not mean we must all stick with the same job. We might find rejuvenation in what Americans call a 'bridge job' – a lateral move to something new. Or in getting back to the shop floor. Older workers' skills that look redundant in one place can be valuable somewhere else: one UK supermarket group is now employing retired business executives from other companies as wine specialists, dealing with customers. They don't mind the drop in status; they enjoy talking to people about their passion.

Manifestly, it is easier to make such transitions if you are senior and well connected. The picture can look very different from the ranks of middle management and junior roles. With the advent of the gig economy, we will need what I am calling start-up trade unions to support people through transitions. Japan's Silver Centres are one unsung model: quietly doing a lot of people a lot of good.

As we head into the Fourth Industrial Revolution, we will need a fourth stage of education to guide us. That fourth stage should build on the latest discoveries about how we learn, which are coming from neuroscience.

5

New Neurons

Old brains can *learn new tricks – and they must, to keep in shape*

DAMN! I'VE HIT THE wrong hawk again. Instead of a tingling burst of feathers on the screen, there's an unforgiving beep.

I'm sitting at my computer, trying to spot birds which flash up intermittently in a blue sky. They are all grey, with outstretched wings, but the one I'm supposed to hit in the flock is slightly darker. As I get better at spotting them, they disappear faster, and I'm clicking my mouse in response to something my eyes have tracked, but I'm barely even aware of.

This is HawkEye, a brain training game. It's not the jolliest I've ever played, but it promises to sharpen up my brain beyond simply getting faster at mouse-clicking. Trials have found that older people who play enough hours of this kind of game have fewer car crashes – and even, apparently, a lower risk of dementia.

'Every week someone will ask me, will I be OK if I do crossword puzzles?' says the bearded neuroscientist Henry Mahncke, CEO of Posit Science, which makes this game. 'My answer is no. Yes, you are thinking – you're trying to find an anagram or a synonym – but you're not making the brain faster or more accurate. For that you need to really challenge yourself.'

There is now a whole industry selling online brain training. So far, the hype has exceeded the science. But in the science lies a kernel of something really important: the newfound knowledge that we are continually remoulding the connections between our brain cells as we experience the world, and that our own behaviour can actually change our brains.

The discovery that our brains keep changing and developing throughout our lives is revolutionary. It should profoundly alter our attitude to ageing.

For years, we believed that the brain cells we were born with were basically a lifetime quota, slowly withering. We thought the brain became fixed in adulthood, so that old dogs couldn't learn new tricks. As a result, we haven't bothered to train older workers. We assume that anyone over 60 who studies Mandarin or French is doing it as a hobby. We think that memory loss is inevitable. We have even been told that our characters are wired to a 'happiness set point' which cannot be changed.

All of this, it turns out, is wrong.

Neuroscientists have long known that from birth our brain cells (neurons) combine what we see, hear, taste, touch and smell with our accumulating stock of memories and experiences. They also knew that these neural connections build on each other, enabling us to learn. But for most of the last century, the orthodoxy was that this 'neuroplasticity' ended with childhood. It was almost impossible to imagine shuffling the deckchairs in an adult brain, with its roughly 100 million neurons making 100 trillion connections.

Look at one of those coloured diagrams of the brain in a school textbook. Different parts of the brain are labelled with the functions they control. 'Taste' might be one, 'memory' another. Brain imaging has even shown us which particular region of the brain can solve a logic puzzle, or spot a familiar face in a crowd. The implication is that if something goes wrong in that region, you'll lose the skill. Yet these simple pictures fail to capture what we now know, in the twenty-first century, is the brain's extraordinary adaptability.

The truth is exhilarating. Brand new neurons have been found even in the brains of 70-year-olds with terminal cancer.[1] People have recovered from strokes, despite permanently damaging whole areas of their brains, because other areas have stepped in, like airline passengers seizing the controls from an unconscious pilot. Scientists are finding new ways to help people with psychiatric disorders over-come their conditions, by calming down certain circuits in the brain and rewiring others. And 70-year-olds are learning second languages (though they won't perfect the accent – that particular window does seem to close at age 10).

If we are to enjoy our Extra Time, we need to extend our mental lifespans to match our physical ones. Neuroscience doesn't have all the answers yet, but it is beginning to provide us with some guide-lines for improving our brains and for approaching our brains in the same way that we now approach our bodies: as systems which we can improve, rather than a mystical organ which controls us.

A Brief History of Neuroplasticity

Today's neuroscientists owe a great deal to the humble canary and to an avid bird-watcher called Fernando Nottebohm. Growing up on a ranch in Argentina, Nottebohm kept birds as pets. He became especially fond of singing birds and wanted to know what they were saying to each other. This led him to make a breakthrough discovery in 1983, which eventually changed the way we think about the brain.

Most birds sing the same songs every year to attract a mate. But Nottebohm noticed that canaries and zebra finches, like hit record producers, would make up entirely new melodies each year.[2] In his lab at Rockefeller University, he examined the brains of these birds and saw that the canaries' brains almost doubled in size every spring, when they were singing, then shrank at the end of the breeding season, when they fell silent. The birds were creating new brain cells – neurons – in the regions of the brain which governed singing and learning.

This phenomenon, the creation of brand-new brain cells in adult brains, is called neurogenesis. Nottebohm's first proofs of neurogenesis were greeted with huge scepticism because neurons, unlike other cells, do not divide. It was later discovered[3] that our brains have a store of neuronal stem cells, which can transform into other cells. But this was not known at the time and many experts dismissed the findings as a peculiarity unique to a few warbling birds.

A decade later, however, scientists had conclusively proved that neurogenesis occurs in adult human brains too: in the hippocampus.[4] Shaped like a horseshoe, the hippocampus is a memory-generating powerhouse which lies deep inside the brain under the cerebral cortex. It enables us to learn new information, consolidate it and stash it away in our long-term memories. Like a vast filing system, it also stores memories of where things are. Without it, we would not be able to remember where we live, or find our keys. The reason why Alzheimer's sufferers find it difficult to remember those things is because Alzheimer's affects the hippocampus first, before any other part of the brain.

The hippocampus grows larger in creatures which need to do a lot of remembering – like squirrels, which hide nuts in summer to dig up in winter, or London taxi drivers, who have to pass 'The Knowledge': a test which requires them to memorise 24,000 streets and 50,000 landmarks within six miles of Charing Cross railway station. A five-year study by Eleanor Maguire and colleagues at University College London found that these taxi drivers had far more grey matter in their posterior (back) hippocampi (the bit which concerns spatial navigation) than average citizens did. And more than London bus drivers,[5] who only have to follow a few set routes.

Maguire's MRI scans proved that people who became taxi drivers hadn't started off with some kind of lopsided brain; it was the actual process of learning the streets which enlarged their hippocampus. In other words, cognitive exercise can produce physical changes in the brain. That has big implications for how we might train our brains as we get older.

Teaching Old Mice New Tricks

At the Salk Institute for Biological Studies, La Jolla, California, Professor Fred 'Rusty' Gage and his colleague Gerd Kempermann created a sort of Disneyland for mice, with wheels, balls, tunnels and lots of other mice to socialise with. They discovered that this dramatically increased the number of new neurons produced in the mouse brains.[6] After 45 days, these mice were generating 15 per cent more new neurons than before – and these new neurons were surviving, not just dying off.

The effects were just as dramatic with older mice. Eighteen-month-old mice, the equivalent of 65-year-old humans, developed five times the number of new neurons in the hippocampus when in the Disneyland environment than in commonplace cages. No matter what age the mice were, the experience was just as rejuvenating for their brains.

The scientists weren't sure which aspects of the enriched experience – hanging out with other mice, trying out new toys, or running on wheels – produced most neurons. It turned out that physical exercise – running round wheels and through tunnels – had by far the biggest effect. Mice in cages with running wheels produced twice as many new neurons as sedentary mice did. Getting active can enlarge our brains, it seems, just as it can build our muscles.

What's more, these mice proved to be better at learning to navigate mazes than those raised in duller conditions. In an unpleasant experiment,[7] mice were dunked in a water tank in which they were out of their depth in all but one area, where there was a submerged platform. The little creatures paddled desperately until their feet hit this platform. In subsequent tests, the wheel-runners were significantly better at remembering where this platform was, and landing on it again.

Other research has found that wheel-running mice develop many more dendrites, the little spikes through which neurons receive signals from each other, than sedentary mice. This could be highly significant, as dendrites are the part of the neuron which tend to deteriorate with age – and affect learning and memory.

Human brains also benefit from aerobic exercise. One group of older people who participated in an aerobic fitness programme for three months were found to have significantly increased their brain volume, while another group who did stretching and toning did not.[8] This is likely to be because aerobic exercise increases the blood supply and oxygen to the hippocampus. Exercise also stimulates production of a protein called brain-derived neurotrophic factor, or BDNF, which is vital for neurogenesis.

Use It or Lose It?

Brains create new neurons all the time, but neurons also die away, half within only a few weeks of their creation. That is what happened in Nottebohm's songbirds, which had a smash hit every spring but ran out of melodies each autumn. Wheel-running mice follow a similar pattern: they produce more new brain cells than sedentary mice, but their brain cells die away at a similar rate.

The best way to sustain these brain cells for longer is to incorporate them into the functional circuits of the brain[9] by learning something new. Gage and his colleagues found that the wheel-running mice who were also living in the enriched environments lost brain cells at a slower rate than those who were just running on wheels in standard cages.[10] While exercise was vital, there was something profound about the combination of physical activity, the pleasure of interacting with other mice and the stimulation of mastering new toys and exploring new environments.

The simple conclusion is that our brains will lack nourishment if we get stuck in a rut. It is now believed that being housebound or in hospital, stuck in one environment, can speed brain atrophy. This makes it even more important to reduce the number of falls and fractures which send people to hospital.

How the Brain Rewires Itself

A child's brain is plastic, learning and forming new memories by making new connections between neurons. But their brain is also plastic in the sense that the actual parts of the brain will change roles according to what the child is doing. When my son learns the violin, for example, his brain allocates more space to the fingers which hold down the strings. We now know that adult brains are plastic too. If you take up a musical instrument at the age of 50, the cortical area of your brain will reorganise itself to support your new skill even if you've never played before.[11]

We know this because modern neuroscientists, like Victorian cartographers, have painstakingly mapped the landscape of the brain. Brain cells are organised in the visual cortex, the somatosensory cortex and the motor cortex to reflect the way that different parts of the body relate to each other. If I touch your thumb, a signal goes through the spinal cord and up to a particular point in your motor cortex, where it turns on cells in the map, which will make you feel your thumb is being touched. The map for the thumb is located next to the map for the index finger, which is next to the map for the middle finger, and so on. If I touch those parts of the map electrically, I can make you feel as though your fingers have been touched.

A young neuroscientist called Michael Merzenich painstakingly mapped some of these connections from the 1970s onwards, by pioneering the use of tiny microelectrodes, which detect when one individual neuron fires off an electrical signal to another. What he discovered – contrary to the colourful pictures in the old textbooks – was that these brain maps vary from person to person, and that they change according to how we live.

Merzenich's most legendary experiment was when he brain-mapped the hand of an adult rhesus monkey, and then amputated the monkey's middle finger.[12] A few months later, he mapped the brain of the long-suffering monkey again. The brain map for the amputated finger had completely disappeared – a striking example of 'use it or lose it'. Its place had been taken by the maps for the next-door fingers, which had grown into the vacated space. The brain had, rapidly and effortlessly, re-allocated its resources to where it could be useful.

Something similar happened when Merzenich took another long-suffering monkey and cut its median nerve. When he stroked the middle of the monkey's hand, the brain map was silent. But when he stroked the outer parts of the hand, served by other nerves, the median nerve part of the map immediately responded. In only a few months, the maps of the other nerves had completely taken over the vacant space.

Learning from Strokes

The finding that maps could rearrange themselves so easily revolutionised the approach to stroke patients. Until the twenty-first century, few believed that radical rehabilitation was possible after stroke, in which a clot in a blood vessel cuts off oxygen to parts of the brain.

Stroke used to kill, but now a majority survive. It is the leading cause of long-term adult disability in the world, affecting 100,000 Brits and 795,000 Americans each year, most of whom end up with some paralysis on one side of the body.[13] One approach has involved making patients spend hours painstakingly trying to move the paralysed hand or arm, while constraining the good hand or arm in a sling, to encourage the brain to recruit new regions to send signals to the paralysed limb. This Constraint-Induced Movement Therapy[14] was pioneered by Edward Taub, who argued that when humans quickly give up on an affected limb, their brain will not grow new neural pathways – in fact may even suppress them. This 'learned non-use' can, however, be overcome by strenuous, repeated attempts to move – and has been remarkably successful in some determined patients.

The very nature of neuroplasticity means that the brain can collude with us in harmful ways, as well as positive ones. Dr Lara Boyd, a brain researcher at the University of British Columbia who works with stroke patients, puts it to me this way: 'Your brain is being shaped by everything you do, but also by what you don't do. Neuroplasticity can be positive – you learn something new – but it can also be negative – you become addicted to drugs, or you have chronic pain.' Dr Boyd believes that 'brain health is a huge issue. I don't think people understand that every little choice is making a difference to their brain. All those little bits add up.'

A major limitation in helping people recover from stroke, Dr Boyd has found, is that patterns of neuroplasticity are highly variable from person to person. Initially, she and her team thought this was unique to stroke sufferers, but they have found similar diver gence in healthy people. This poses a real challenge for helping people learn.

'We learn in highly unique ways,' she says. 'When two people are trying to learn the same task, we can see it in different patterns of brain activity: the circuits they are using and the intensity. Let's say you and I are trying to learn to move a limb. You may just use the motor areas of your brain. But I can only do it if I continue to use more cognitive areas of the brain, which deal with executive function.' There's a penalty, she says, to using those additional systems: 'I might become as proficient as you, but if I try to do something else at the same time, I may not be able to.'

Boyd says that her father-in-law, an otherwise healthy 86-year-old, is a good example of the way in which one part of the brain can inhibit another. 'He can't walk and talk at the same time,' she explains. 'We'll be talking and I suddenly think, "Where did he go?" He has stopped walking, in order to talk. He doesn't realise he's doing it.'

As a result of these differences, she is sceptical about the fashionable thesis that it takes 10,000 hours to master any new motor skill. 'It might take *you* 5,000 hours, but it might take *me* 20,000,' she says.

Recognising that we are all different, Boyd and her colleagues are now trying to develop therapies which can 'prime' the brain to learn. 'You're never too old to learn,' she says. 'There's no drug you can take – the primary driver of neuroplastic change in your brain is your own behaviour. But the dose needed to learn new skills, or relearn old ones, is very large.' She advocates 'increased struggles' which lead to more learning and to structural change in the brain, which underpins long-term memories.

Dr Boyd's work makes a strong argument for tailoring treatment to the individual. Eventually, she hopes, stroke will be treated like cancer: using biomarkers[15] of brain structure to create individualised patient plans, just as doctors now use genetics to devise personalised regimes of chemotherapy. It also suggests that the most effective teaching will be personalised. 'The uniqueness of your brain will affect you as a learner or teacher,' says Boyd. 'Each of us will need to do something different – that's the next frontier of neuroscience.'

'Neurons That Fire Together, Wire Together'

One thing which has puzzled me is why we don't run out of map space. If we take up a new pursuit, or we regain the use of a hand,

and our brain devotes more space to that, why doesn't this diminish some other ability? There may indeed be trade-offs, as researchers speculated when they looked at London taxi drivers (see pages 104–5). But the main reason we don't swamp the grey matter is that the more we train ourselves to do something, the more efficiently our neurons work together.

Bill Jenkins, a behavioural psychologist who worked with Michael Merzenich, trained monkeys to touch a spinning disc with their fingertips, giving them a banana pellet reward if they could exert the right amount of pressure to keep it spinning. This was tricky: the monkeys had to concentrate hard. But the brains of those who worked at it grew steadily, in the area which mapped their fingertip. The more they tried, the more their brains responded. After a certain point, each neuron within the map became more effective and eventually, fewer neurons were required to succeed in keeping the disc spinning.[16]

Something similar happens when a human learns a new trick, say juggling. If we repeatedly use our fingers in a way which requires intense focus and sensitivity, the individual neurons will eventually start to fire faster. Neurons which fire faster are more likely to fire in sync with each other and to give out clearer signals.

This is very important, because clearer signals improve memory. One reason we forget things as we get older, scientists now believe, is that our brains are struggling through 'noise': fuzzy signals given out by neurons which are not syncing properly. We process new events more slowly as we get older, which makes it harder to form a clear memory of someone's name, or who said what at the party.

Many scientists are now trying to find ways to reduce the 'noise' in our brains as we age. One way is challenging ourselves in ways which require our full attention. When monkeys perform tasks on autopilot, or are distracted, their brain maps alter slightly, but the changes do not persist.

The Power of Music

What should we do, to challenge our brains? Two activities which require an intense focus, where there has been robust research, are learning a foreign language and playing a musical instrument. Musicians who practise regularly and intensively have been found to have more grey matter in part of their frontal lobe, and less age-related degeneration in other parts of the brain, than non-musicians.[17] One group of people over 75 who frequently played a musical instrument were found to be less likely to have developed dementia after five years than those who rarely played.[18] The protective effect of playing music was found to be stronger than reading, writing or doing puzzles.[19]

Crossword puzzles have had a good press. Some studies show that people who do crosswords have better cognitive function than those who don't.[20] Unfortunately, this proves only that clever people enjoy crosswords. Puzzlers seem to suffer cognitive decline at the same rate as non-puzzlers. So crosswords probably won't protect us from decline.

Frankly, this is all a bit exhausting. It suggests that slumping into a comfortable middle age, drinking with friends and chairing the same old committee may be storing up trouble. Conversely, it suggests that we may be able to improve our learning and speed of memory if we do things which inspire a virtuous cycle of brain plasticity.

How 'Cognitive Reserve' May Protect Against Alzheimer's

In his book *Aging with Grace*,[21] the American epidemiologist David Snowdon describes the moment when he and his team realised that an 85-year-old nun, Sister Bernadette, had been functioning perfectly up until her death, despite having full-blown Alzheimer's in her brain.

Analysis of Sister Bernadette's brain tissue found the tangles and plaques which indicate Alzheimer's. But she had been achieving normal scores on all of the mental and physical tests the researchers had given her. In a particularly impressive videotaped exchange done with each exam, Sister Bernadette – without looking at a clock or a watch – had stated the time within four minutes of the actual time. Sister Bernadette had a Master's degree. She had taught at elementary school for 21 years and at high school for another seven. Her brain function seemed to be incredibly preserved, Snowdon remembered. 'It was as if her neocortex was resistant to destruction.'

The idea that some brains could be resistant to destruction, even in very old age, had not even occurred to David Snowdon when he founded the 'Nun Study': with 1,200 Catholic nuns in holy orders across the US. These wonderful ladies agreed to complete physical and cognitive tests every year, and to donate their brains after death. They made an ideal control group: they were all white, ate the same food, lived in the same places for decades, and didn't drink or smoke or get pregnant. Their act of generosity, in leaving their brains to science, reaped earthly rewards which are still flowing.

Snowdon was, by his own account, inappropriately excited when he received the first brain, in a UPS package. 'Remember, somebody died,' a colleague admonished him. As he accumulated brains, he discovered something extraordinary. Nearly a third of the brains tested at autopsy showed signs of full-blown Alzheimer's. But not all of the owners of those brains showed symptoms.[22] Some continued to pass cognitive tests with flying colours, well into their eighties and nineties.

Incredibly, the strongest predictor of who would suffer the symptoms of Alzheimer's turned out to be the quality of autobiographical essays the nuns had written at the age of 22, when they took their final vows. An astonishing 90 per cent of the women who later developed Alzheimer's had written essays with what the researchers called 'low idea density' – relatively few ideas expressed in every ten words – and low grammatical complexity. Of those whose writing was more idea-dense and complex, only 13 per cent developed the disease.[23]

Idea density reflects language processing capacity, which is associated with a person's level of education, general knowledge, vocabulary and reading comprehension. Grammatical complexity is associated with working memory, which helps us keep different elements in play and not lose our train of thought.

'Cognitive reserve' is the brain's ability to improvise: its plasticity. Other research has confirmed Snowdon's findings that cognitive reserve is correlated with higher levels of education.[24] This doesn't mean a professor can't get Alzheimer's, but it does suggest that brains which are plastic may be able to re-order themselves to resist its ravages for longer. Studies have suggested that people with higher cognitive reserve may be better at staving off Parkinson's disease and stroke, as well as dementia.[25]

Highly educated people should be thankful – for both their good luck in their upbringing, and to the nuns for selflessly donating their brains. But we can all read to our children, to stimulate their language development. And we can all work at keeping our brain cells active. Harvard Medical School has developed a six-step programme for cognitive health.[26] The tenets are: eat a plant-based diet, exercise regularly, get enough sleep, manage stress, nurture social contacts and keep challenging your brain.

But how should we, realistically, challenge our brains? Not everyone has an aptitude for music. Not everyone can face learning a language – especially if they know they'll have no chance to use it. This is one reason for the growing popularity of brain-training apps.

Should You Buy a Brain-Training App?

The brain-training game I played at the beginning of this chapter is one of a burgeoning number, in an industry rumoured to be worth almost $1 billion. Many firms now offer games to people who want to stay mentally alert. Cognifit tests 23 different cognitive skills and provides 'personalized brain games' to 'help stimulate cognitive functions and improve brain plasticity'. HAPPYneuron offers 'a complete brain training method to stimulate the 5 main cognitive functions'. Nintendo is currently marketing a video game called Brain Age 2.

Most apps claim that daily practice will improve your brain's ability not only to hit the target, or to memorise a sequence of numbers as they flash past, but also to get mentally sharper in real life. It's wise to view these claims with some scepticism. In 2016, a company called Lumosity.com agreed to pay a $50 million settlement to the Federal Trade Commission over claims of false advertising, which the FTC said had 'preyed on consumers' fears about age-related cognitive decline'. Lumosity, it said, did not have proven scientific evidence to back its claims that its games could improve performance at work and ward off memory loss and dementia. The FTC agreed that Lumosity's games might improve your skill at playing that particular game, but not that doing so necessarily improves your ability to remember who you met last night or find your wallet.[27]

Some of the world's leading cognitive psychologists and neuroscientists expressed similar concerns in 2014, at a meeting convened by the Stanford Center on Longevity and the Berlin Max Planck Institute for Human Development.[28] The 69 experts published a joint statement condemning hype and saying that gains made through brain-training apps often lapse. 'Any mentally effortful new experience, such as learning a language, acquiring a motor skill, navigating in a new environment, and, yes, playing commercially available computer games, will produce changes in those neural systems that support acquisition of the new skill,' they wrote. 'There may be an increase in the number of synapses, the number of neurons and supporting cells, or a strengthening of the connections among them ... however at this point it is not appropriate to conclude that training-induced changes go significantly beyond the learned skills, that they affect broad abilities with real-world relevance, or that they generally promote "brain health".'[29]

The group also worried that people might spend weeks sitting at screens, rather than doing something healthy. 'If an hour spent doing solo software drills is an hour not spent hiking, learning Italian, making a new recipe, or playing with your grandchildren, it may not be worth it,' they wrote.

A few months later, however, a group of 133 international scientists and practitioners expressed a very different view. A 'substantial and growing body of evidence,' they said, 'shows that certain cognitive training regimens can significantly improve cognitive function, including in ways that generalize to everyday life.'[30]

Why did these two groups disagree so starkly? Partly because lumping together all brain training games makes no sense. Much of what's on the market is unproven. A 2016 review of every scientific paper cited by brain training companies found that many were woefully flawed: with tiny sample sizes or no control groups.[31] There's also the 'file drawer problem': research which shows no benefit doesn't get published. But a few trials do give reason for hope, in some very specific areas.

The game I was playing at the beginning of this chapter is meant to improve 'speed processing'. Also called useful field of view (UFOV) training, this is designed to improve how fast and accurately your brain processes what you see. The computer forces you to divide your attention between objects at the centre of the screen and targets on the periphery. As you get better at the game, the targets become obscured in a blizzard of other objects, forcing you to work harder to stay focused.

A ten-year trial, ACTIVE,[32] claimed to have found lasting cognitive improvements in those who played speed-processing games compared with those who didn't, including those who spent time in other kinds of training. The researchers divided the 2,800 volunteers, aged between 65 and 94, into three groups. The first were given strategies to improve memory, the second strategies to improve reasoning, and the third received individualised computer training on speed of processing.

Volunteers who trained their brain speed got better at remembering to take their medications, and doing things which required attention, like preparing meals. They also reported being in a better mood. But even more striking was what happened to their driving. ACTIVE volunteers who trained their brain speed were half as likely to experience a car crash as those who had not trained. Forty per cent fewer people in that group gave up driving. And their insurance claims dropped by a quarter from what they had been before. It looks as though having a faster processing speed could make the difference between hitting a cyclist and stopping in time.

ACTIVE has its critics. Dan Simons, the psychologist whose team reviewed the scientific studies,[33] says that the ACTIVE trial stood out as rigorous, but it doesn't prove that online games have real-world effects. 'The things you train will improve, but they don't generalize,' Simons told *The Atlantic*.[34] 'If you search baggage scans for a knife, you don't get better at spotting guns.'

There is a heated debate about how high the bar should be. When you play the piano, you don't get better at soccer, but we still think that playing piano is good for your brain. Speed processing doesn't seem to improve memory, but if it improves driving and keeps elderly people on the road safely for longer, that's a benefit.

'Many people are sceptical that 10–12 hours of brain training can have lasting real-world effects,' says Alvaro Fernandez, an ebullient Spaniard who runs SharpBrains, an independent consultancy tracking brain research in Washington, DC. 'But ACTIVE showed a clear impact on driving safety: what better transfer can you have to the real world? In any case, the average old person watches TV for four to five hours a day, why not do some brain training instead?'

Professor Jerri Edwards, of the University of South Florida, which oversaw ACTIVE, says, 'UFOV training is a particularly promising approach. One reason is that this training technique typically includes exercises that are adaptive in difficulty. The model of adult plasticity indicates that cognitive training programmes that are adaptive in difficulty will be most effective.'

Adaptive games evolve so that your brain continues to be challenged, keeping the intense focus that Michael Merzenich and others say is so vital. Merzenich is the founder of Posit Science, which makes the UFOV training used in ACTIVE. Notwithstanding the fact that he now has a commercial interest, which everyone should be aware of, I'm inclined to think he may be on to something, given his track record.

The most recent finding from the ACTIVE trial is that UFOV training may reduce the incidence of dementia.[35] Volunteers who completed at least ten hours of that training were 29 per cent less likely to get dementia than those in the control groups. The more computerised sessions they completed, the more their risk fell.

These figures are not overwhelming. The risk of getting dementia in the control groups was only 11 per cent. And no one is claiming that a computer programme can treat dementia, once someone has got it. Nevertheless, it does suggest that UFOV training might improve the brain's resilience.

The NHS and other health services should now be looking at this kind of brain training, in my view. When the US National Academies of Science, Engineering and Medicine examined 17 possible ways to slow cognitive decline and dementia, it concluded the three most promising were physical activity, blood pressure management and cognitive training, including speed-processing programmes.[36] It also declared that none of these were backed by sufficiently strong evidence – yet – to launch a public campaign. But the evidence is growing for all three, especially if cognitive training is defined as UFOV training.

Tackling Depression: What I Wish I'd Known to Help My Father

My father's later years were overshadowed by crippling black moods. Physically fit and healthy into his late eighties, with hearing so good he sometimes wished for a little deafness when the pub opposite his house held a band night, he suffered bouts of depression which could make him feel physically ill. 'There's something in my brain that just doesn't want me to be happy,' he'd reflect sadly. He was usually one of the most cheerful, optimistic people I knew, but as he grew older he couldn't seem to stop going over sad stories in the newspaper and over-analysing chance remarks made by friends.

Depression is set to be the single biggest cause of disability worldwide in the next 20 years.[37] If we are to make the most of Extra Time, we need to take it much more seriously. The Royal College of Psychiatrists says that almost nine out of ten elderly people with depression get no help, because doctors struggle to spot the symptoms or confuse it with dementia. In addition, many older people assume that depression is just part of ageing, so don't even seek help. Bereavement is miserable. Loneliness must be tackled. But depression is not a normal part of ageing.

My father did seek help, but antidepressants just made him feel sick. He stopped going to parties. He didn't want to see anyone but his closest friends and relatives. He stopped driving, with great regret, when he realised his failing eyesight was a danger to others. His world shrank.

My breezy remedy was to encourage him to get out and exercise, which always improves my own mood. I tried to persuade him to come for walks. But he was brilliantly evasive, allergic to the idea of 'fitness' and convinced that his daily stroll to the newsagent was quite enough.

I now realise that he was, perhaps, more right than we both knew: there really was something in his brain that didn't want him to enjoy life. Depression is often associated with entrenched patterns of thought. Some psychiatrists now believe that these patterns translate into brain circuits, which are more easily triggered the more times they are used.

It may be possible to form new neural connections to reset such patterns. Mindfulness training programmes, such as that pioneered by Jon Kabat-Zinn, aim to reduce stress by teaching people to become more aware of their thoughts and to see negative thoughts as only fleeting, temporary. Some therapists, like John Teasdale at Cambridge University, have used mindfulness cognitive therapy to dramatically reduce the risk of relapse in depressed participants.[38] Brain scans show that CBT dampens down activity in the frontal cortex, the seat of reasoning and higher thought – reducing our tendency to dwell on the bad. And it increases activity in the hippocampus, perhaps forming new, more positive, patterns of thought.[39]

Could meditation beat medication? Some scientists believe that some kinds of meditation, practised regularly, can reduce stress and improve concentration. One study asked eight Tibetan Buddhist monks and ten college students to meditate, and compared their brain waves.[40] The monks achieved strong gamma frequencies, which are thought to promote synchronised firing of neurons. Another study of 13 Zen practitioners found that they had far less decline in grey matter and better reaction times than the control group.[41] Frankly, there isn't enough proof yet – and the definition of 'meditation' is probably too broad. But the coming decade may shed more light.

Not only does depression cause utter misery, it can also impair our ability to think.[42] It can impact on memory, information-processing and decision-making skills. Antidepressants which improve mood don't always tackle these cognitive factors, according to some experts, who argue that greater attention should be paid to helping people keep functioning.

The Theory of Inflammation

In 1989, Edward Bullmore was 29 and was training as a physician just before he started to specialise in psychiatry. In walked a patient, Mrs P, in her late fifties. Mrs P suffered from severe rheumatoid arthritis, a painful autoimmune disease. The swelling in her hands was terrible: Bullmore could see that her fingers were distorted and the joints disfigured by scarring. He talked her through her physical symptoms, which ticked the box for rheumatoid arthritis. Then he departed from convention and asked about her state of mind. Mrs P unloaded. She explained that she had very low levels of energy, couldn't take pleasure in anything and was sleeping badly. He concluded that she was clinically depressed.

'I was quite excited,' Bullmore recalls slightly sheepishly. 'I felt I'd made a minor medical discovery. I thought, I've doubled her diagnosis – she came in thinking she only had arthritis, and I've turned her into a patient with arthritis and depression.'

He rushed to his boss with the news – who just shrugged. 'Well, you'd be depressed, wouldn't you? If you had that disability and you knew it was only going to get worse?'

At the time, the conventional medical view was that depression was all in the mind. It did not occur to Bullmore that Mrs P's depression might originate in the body. It was not until much later that he began to wonder if the depression could in fact be related to the inflammation which was causing her arthritis.

Now Professor of Psychiatry at the University of Cambridge and author of *The Inflamed Mind*,[43] Bullmore is one of the leaders in the new field of neuroimmunology, which draws connections between the brain and the immune system.

At its most basic, inflammation in the body is a response to infection. If you cut your finger, a type of white blood cell called a macrophage will eat up harmful bacteria like a Pac-Man and pump out cytokines, inflammatory proteins which tell the rest of the immune system there is an infection. Swelling and tenderness are the usual result, as other macrophages rush to the site.

When inflammation goes awry, in autoimmune disorders like rheumatoid arthritis, the swelling and tenderness can become permanent features. In this case the immune system has overreacted and turned against the body. Type 2 diabetes, cancer, Parkinson's and Alzheimer's have all been linked to this kind of 'inflammaging', which has got out of control.

This is a particular problem as we age. Our immune systems weaken and we become more vulnerable to infection. That's why vaccinations often don't work in older people. The immune system can misfire, targeting the wrong things.

Practising as a psychiatrist, Bullmore found himself seeing many patients like Mrs P. 'I kept thinking: so many patients with inflammatory disorders have depression, why can't we do a better job?' he says. Antidepressant SSRIs like Prozac work for many people, especially alongside therapy. But not for everyone. And they can have side effects. Despite billions of pounds worth of investment by pharmaceutical companies, no significant new antidepressant drugs have come to market since Prozac, 28 years ago. Bullmore began to wonder if they were looking in the wrong place. And if the blood-brain barrier, a membrane which protects the brain from toxins in the blood, might be more permeable than anyone thought.

It now appears that certain signals from the blood can cause mischief in the brain, exciting immune cells and stirring up inflammation.

Our immune systems are exquisitely responsive to the outside world. Stresses of all kinds cause low-grade inflammation in the blood: in burned-out teachers, or people caring for sick relatives, or traumatised children. This is also true of rats. If young rats are restrained, or removed from their mothers, they exhibit classic signs of depression. They behave in a similar way, Bullmore says, if they are injected with cytokines. This activates immune cells in the brain.

'The immune system has a phenomenal memory,' says Bullmore. 'If you were exposed to measles as a child, your immune system will remember that till the day you die. Could it not be that our immune systems respond to social threats in the same way?

'You can see changes in how the neurons work,' he adds. 'They are less plastic and more likely to die.'

When rats are restrained in small cages, neurogenesis slows almost to a halt.[44] You would assume that it's depression which is dampening the creation of new neurons. In fact, it may be the other way around.

There is no conclusive proof that anti-inflammatory treatments curb depression. Further research is needed. But these discoveries make it possible that the next great strides in combating depression may be made by neuroscientists who are working on inflammation and neurogenesis: offering up the possibility that what happens in the body could be intimately connected with what happens in the mind.

What If Older People Can Learn, But They Learn Differently to Younger Ones?

When Zoe Kourtzi was a teenager growing up in Crete, she had a terrible memory for facts. 'History was a killer,' she laughs, her dark eyes crinkling at the memory. 'There are so many dates in Greece. When people were born, when they died; it's such an ancient civilisation.' Now Professor of Experimental Psychology at Cambridge University, Zoe had to pass History, Maths and Ancient Greek to be accepted to study Psychology, which she had set her heart on, despite her mother's suggestion that she be a hairdresser. She knew she could pass Maths, her favourite subject. But to pass History and Ancient Greek, she needed a strategy. In desperation, she tape-recorded herself reading out key historical dates and Greek vocabulary and played the tapes back every night.

She passed her exams and 'wiped them from my memory the next day'. But along the way she had discovered something. While History required her to memorise facts, Ancient Greek felt more like Maths: 'I realised that Greek was really a logic problem. To learn a language, you have to be able to interpret and understand the structure of language.'

Our school systems are obsessed with learning by rote. And we adults are paranoid about memory loss. But what if being able to decipher patterns turns out to be almost as useful, for functioning in the real world, as memorising?

Nowadays, Kourtzi presides over the Adaptive Brain Lab at Cambridge. It's in a jumble of 1950s and Gothic buildings, concealed behind the Palladian purity of Downing College. Inside the Lab, there's a striking illusion on the wall. It's a picture of a Venice canal, but the buildings seem to jut out from the wall.

'Run your finger over it,' Kourtzi says, bouncing over to the wall. 'Can you feel it's indented?' Running my hand over the picture, I can feel that the picture has raised parts and indented parts. But the grand palazzo buildings which I think are closest are actually farthest away.

My brain refuses to go along with what my fingers tell me. Knowing the picture's shape is the opposite of what I thought doesn't change the way I see it. 'Why I can't I see it right?' I ask in frustration. 'Because a lifetime of experience is more important to your brain than what I tell you,' says Professor Kourtzi, smiling. 'What falls on your retina is not what your brain perceives. It knows that when squares are larger, they are generally closer to you. So that's the way it perceives them.'

Similarly, she says, when people are put into an MRI scanner and shown a static picture of an athlete at the start line of a race, the part of their brain associated with motion lights up. We expect motion, so we neurologically 'see' it, even though the athlete is standing still.

Kourtzi's team are trying to unravel the mechanisms which underlie how brains learn. The lab is full of screens on which the team are training different age groups to decipher objects in cluttered scenes. This kind of visual perception is highly trainable – it's how we spot a face in a crowd. In the Second World War, Allied military analysts poring over grainy aerial reconnaissance photos gradually got better and better at being able to tell the difference between a camouflaged V-weapon, for example, and an innocuous pylon.

As someone struggles their way through cascading coloured dots and other moving images, the team will scan their brains to see what is happening to their brain circuits. They have made several fascinating discoveries.

First, it appears that age is no bar to learning. What matters more is the way you learn and your attitude. 'If older people have really good attentive abilities,' Kourtzi explains, 'they can learn as fast as younger ones.' There are strong learners and weak learners in all age groups, she says.

Strong learners are those who can attend to multiple things at the same time and recruit the areas of the brain which are involved in attention. Weak learners rely more on memory, 'which we can see from greater activity in those parts of the brain'. This may explain why human memory is fallible: we don't actually need to remember every image because what our brains are doing is trying to generalise from them. To function well in later life, memory may be less important than being able to multi-task and spot patterns.

The Adaptive Brain Lab has created an artificial 'alien' language, made up of symbols. Participants are asked to predict which symbols should come next in a sequence. Those who try to memorise the symbol order fare markedly worse than those who focus on the rules and structure of the new language. Like the younger Zoe, that dark-haired teenager in Crete, the most successful learners use judgements of probability, not memory.

Kourtzi has also found that older people use different brain circuits from younger people. The young use parts of the anterior brain, associated with perception. The old tend to use posterior parts of the brain, which decipher patterns.

'The clear implication,' she argues, 'is that training programmes need to be geared for age.'

This idea has revolutionary potential. As I wrote in the last chapter, we have barely started thinking about how to help people acquire new skills over the course of a lifetime. And we certainly haven't thought about the fact that different age groups might learn in different ways. But it looks like we need to.

The Future: The Annual Brain Check-Up and AI

'Brain health' is a phrase I've heard repeatedly on my travels, from experts who believe the brain is a system we need to take care of, just as we look after our bodies. Dr Mike Roizen, Chief Wellness Officer at the Cleveland Clinic, summed up a growing view when he said recently that 'the brain may really be like a muscle, and able to get stronger throughout life'.

This is a long way from our usual concept of the brain as a mystical centre of our being, where our personality resides. It's quite hard to get your head around the idea that we could actively change our brains using willpower. But that idea is definitely coming.

'The best analogy is to the fitness movement,' says Alvaro Fernandez of SharpBrains. 'We went from having the general idea of fitness to having gyms, personal trainers and precise exercises. If I want to get stronger abs, I do sit-ups. If I want to be a better all-round athlete, I lift weights. The same will happen with the brain, but it will happen faster because the toolkit is mostly online, and almost everyone has access.'

Mr Fernandez believes we should get annual brain check-ups. Not MRI scans, which would be prohibitively expensive, but cognitive tests, which he expects will become increasingly sophisticated in detecting small changes. AI has huge potential here. Machine-learning algorithims can track patterns which may be able to spot incipient dementia, for example, long before it causes visible symptoms like memory loss. There are already systems which can detect tiny changes in the way we type: how long it takes us to move between the keys, or how long we hold each key down. The Californian company NeuraMatrix believes that its Typing Cadence system could alert users to brain disorders far earlier than any doctor – by picking up changes in typing of only one hundredth of a second.[45] Even more ambitious, MIT researchers have recently recorded the sleep patterns, breathing and movements of people in an assisted-living facility, to see if algorithms can use sleep disturbances and other tiny changes in behaviour to diagnose Alzheimer's.

This matters because the fight against dementia is shifting to earlier diagnosis, with researchers hoping to develop drugs to slow the disease. But they can only do that if they can identify it early enough, and pick out the right patients to recruit for clinical trials.

For many neuroscientists, comparing the brain to a muscle is something of a profanity. But it is a useful analogy in one particular way. I use my bicep muscle every time I lift my forearm. Using it stops it wasting away. But to strengthen it, I need to lift heavy weights, preferably three times a week – and I need to do that systematically before I'll see any results.

The same, it seems, is true of the brain: only regular heavy-lifting produces lasting improvements. Torkel Klingberg, Professor of Cognitive Neuroscience at Stockholm's Karolinska Institute, has described what he has called the 'cognitive gym'.[46] His team has done extensive work to help improve the working memory of children with ADHD and has also trained sixty-somethings to improve working memory. They have seen far stronger effects when people carry out stretching tasks on a daily basis.

What all of this means, I'm afraid, is that we can't afford to slump into a contented middle age.

Teaching 'Young-Old' Dogs New Tricks

Not so long ago, people thought that boys were naturally better than girls at science. We may be making a similar mistake when we assume that older people can't learn as well as younger ones.

The battle to prove that the brain is eternally plastic has been waged for decades, but it's only been comprehensively won in the past ten years. Many people still don't understand the enormous potential of their brains.

We know that brain cells need to stay active to maintain their connections with other neurons. These connections, the synapses, disintegrate and disappear if a cell does not use them to communicate. But there are ways to stave off decline. Aerobic exercise, social contact and new challenges seem to be vital. Playing the same Chopin nocturne for 20 years, as I've been doing, will not cut it. Nor will doing crossword puzzles. We need to maintain our curiosity, and venture into new areas beyond our comfort zone.

The 2017 Lancet Commission on Dementia found that 'physical exercise and intellectual stimulation over the lifespan is associated with reduced risk of dementia in later life, even among individuals with genetic predisposition to dementia'.[47] Yet few adults are even aware that it's possible to reduce the risk of dementia, compared with over three-quarters who recognise that we can reduce our risk of heart disease.[48]

In an area as complex as this, false claims are bound to be made. The marketplace will become increasingly crowded with programmes offering to improve our cognition, not all of which will deliver. But UFOV training does seem to offer genuine hope, and should be looked at by health services.

The great news is that age does not have to be a barrier to learning. Old brains can learn new tricks – and it seems they must, if we are to keep them in shape.

6

In the Genes

*Immortality isn't here yet, but anti-ageing
drugs are on the way*

THIRTY YEARS AGO, DOCTORS assumed that ageing was just something which happened to all of us, and there was nothing we could do about it. But then a handful of pioneering biologists began to identify genes that seemed to influence ageing, and might even postpone it.

Huddling in an unfashionable corner of science, while conventional medicine doggedly continued to treat the sick, these biologists were ignored for a long time. But now their discoveries have taken us to a breakthrough point, where we are about to see a stream of therapies promising to prolong and improve life. Laboratories have doubled the lifespan of worms and made mice and monkeys younger for longer. Quite a few scientists, and even some business executives, are now following regimes which they believe can make them younger.

Some of these scientists are part of the gold rush for immortality: Silicon Valley's quest for 'escape velocity' from death. Others are trying to achieve something even more vital: to reduce the amount of time we spend as 'Old-Old', in frailty at the end of life.

Not all of the products I describe in this chapter will work. There is no single magic bullet, because we probably age along a number of different pathways simultaneously, and the science is complex. But the discoveries are driving a revolution in how ageing is seen, with some scientists arguing that ageing is a disease which can be treated, not something we should passively accept. That has potentially profound consequences for research, regulation and investment – and what products may eventually become available to all of us.

Calorie Restriction – Dangerous Fad or Elixir of Youth?

My friend Antoine, the film producer, is looking gaunt. He's also being remarkably picky over the menu at the restaurant we're in, eventually selecting a fish starter 'as a main', with a side order of kale.

Over the non-existent pudding (Antoine sips at a green tea while I order a full-throated cappuccino), he reveals that he is doing 'CR', as calorie restriction is known to its cult followers in Silicon Valley. For two years, he has tried to eat no more than 1,800 calories a day, 700 below the recommended daily allowance for a man of his height and age. Antoine claims he feels great, clear-minded and energetic. And he believes that this very limited diet could bring him many more years of healthy life.

Experiments since the 1930s have shown that the lifespan of many mammals can be extended by drastically reducing what they eat. Rodents outlive their peers when they are fed only 30–40 per cent of the calories they would normally consume. And they are healthier. They suffer less from cancer, heart disease or cognitive decline.

Remember the Okinawans – the islanders who live to enormously old ages in the far north of Japan? Their philosophy is to eat until they feel about 80 per cent full, and then stop.[1] They call this '*hara hachi bu*' (belly eight parts full). Not only does it do them no harm, it may also be one reason why they have much longer, healthier periods of being 'Young-Old', and much shorter periods of being 'Old-Old', than we Westerners do.

You would think that such drastic dieting would make organisms weak and vulnerable. In fact, it seems to make mice and monkeys stronger (though not necessarily happier – we can't ask them). The theory is that the genes evolved as a response to periods of drought or famine, because individuals who possessed the trait would survive to reproduce. Harsh circumstances set off ancient circuits which protect our cells, and the 'mitochondria' in cells which produce energy.

These circuits are thought to be universal in all animals, including humans. In 2018, researchers published a study of rhesus monkeys, which have human-like ageing patterns.[2] One monkey called Canto started on a 30 per cent calorie restriction diet when he was 16, which for rhesus monkeys is late middle age. He is now 43, the human equivalent of 130.

Could CR be an elixir of youth for humans too? My friend Antoine certainly thinks so, but he looks terribly pale. Extreme calorie restriction is inhuman, basically. It can do terrible things to our bone density and muscle mass; it can impair growth in anyone under 21, and be disastrous for any woman trying to conceive. As a result, it is definitely not recommended by doctors. It's also really difficult to withstand the hunger pangs for any length of time. Since lunching with Antoine, I have met two Silicon Valley entrepreneurs who are doing 'CR' – they talk as if it's a secret code. One admits that he quite often wakes up in the night with hunger pangs and scoffs hard-boiled eggs from the fridge.

Something similar happened when the gerontologist Valter Longo tried to replicate CR by getting his subjects to fast for five consecutive days a month, in an experiment at the University of Southern California.[3] Those who managed this did seem to be healthier, with improved cholesterol and glucose levels. But a quarter of participants couldn't stand it, and dropped out.

I doubt most of us would be prepared to trade the joy of food, even for longer life. So scientists have been looking for ways to trick our bodies into activating those ancient circuits, without us having to go hungry. And they think they've found something.

The Race for the Anti-Ageing Pill

A small grey box has been delivered to my office. 'Elysium Health' it says on the outside in discreet white letters. Inside is a pill bottle containing 60 capsules, my month's supply for which I have paid $60 online.

This is Basis, billed as the 'world's first cellular health product informed by genomics'. This little capsule could, just possibly, give me more years of healthy life.

Basis is sold as a supplement in America, like a vitamin, so it needs no prescription and does not require approval from the US regulator, the Food and Drug Administration (FDA). But it does have an unusually impressive pedigree. There are six Nobel Prize winners on the scientific advisory board of Elysium Health. The pill is the creation of Professor Leonard P. Guarente, the biologist who has made some of the world's most important discoveries about longevity genes over the past 30 years.

I visit Professor Guarente at the Paul F. Glenn Center for Biology of Aging Research that he heads at MIT. It's a huge lab, in a towering glass and sandstone building. I trudge down a long grey corridor lined with huge silver tanks, some marked 'nitrogen', others marked 'cryogenics', past rooms where earnest young men in sweaters hunch over strange-looking machines. In a corner office adorned with stacks of books and a profusion of family photographs, 'Lenny' springs up to greet me. Does he look 64? It's hard to tell. Balding, but spry, in a check shirt and faded jeans, kind eyes twinkling owlishly behind rimless spectacles, he could be younger or older.

Professor Guarente says he's been taking Basis 'longer than anybody – a number of us here started taking it before we launched Elysium' (in 2016). 'How do you know it works?' You're not going to see any immediate results if it's not directly curing anything, just helping people stay the same for longer. He agrees this is a challenge.

'Some people say they have more energy on it,' he says, shrugging. 'But we don't really know. I myself notice that my fingernails grow faster – that's something other people notice too.'

Professor Guarente is remarkably humble about his creation but he is very confident of the science. And he has reason to be. For his journey to this point is an amazing story.

In the 1990s, Guarente had just got divorced and was going through what he calls, sheepishly, 'a bit of a mid-life thing'. Already a tenured professor, he decided to break out from traditional molecular biology into the unconventional backwater of longevity research. He and his team started experimenting on yeast, the simple fungus used to make bread rise. Back then, the idea that yeast could tell us anything about humans seemed totally outlandish. But it turned out that it did.

Guarente and his team found a mutant strain of yeast which had been forgotten in the fridge, but had survived, despite the cold and lack of nourishment. In fact, it ended up living almost 50 per cent longer than other strains, which had endured a less stressful environment.

The answer turned out to lie in a class of genes called sirtuins. When sirtuins are more active, in yeast or in animals, it increases their lifespan. They seem to work by slowing down the progressive accumulation of broken strands of DNA, which build up in all organisms as they age and eventually kill them. The discovery was revolutionary in two ways. First, it proved that there are genes for ageing. Second, it showed that these genes can be manipulated.

In order to function, sirtuins need a wonder molecule, a co-enzyme called NAD+ (nicotinamide adenine dinucleotide). NAD+ drives energy in the body, helps to metabolise food, and maintains healthy DNA. But it declines as we age. By the time we are 50, we have lost around half of our NAD+. And that matters. Studies suggest that boosting levels of NAD+ in older mice can make them look and act younger, and reverse decline in our stem cells[4] – the powerful cells which can replace others in the body as they wear out.

Basis is intended to work the same way, to reverse the decline in NAD+ by activating sirtuins. It contains pterostilbene, found in blueberries and red wine, and nicotinamide riboside, which converts to NAD+ in the body.

At the end of 2017, Elysium published the results of its first randomised, controlled, human trial.[5] One hundred and twenty people aged between 60 and 80 who took Basis for at least four weeks saw an average 40 per cent increase in NAD+ levels. There were, the researchers claim, no harmful side effects.

Guarente is pleased: 'Basis might not have worked, it might not have done in humans what it does in animals. But the trial was testing safety and ability to raise NAD+ levels sustainably, which it did.'

The problem remains that Basis is not an approved medicine. Before the trial, it was attacked as having 'plausible but unproven benefit'.[6] As a supplement, it could be a con. Guarente, it turns out, is scathing about most supplements himself. 'Almost everything in a health and food store doesn't really do anything,' he says. He himself takes Vitamin D in high doses, for which 'there is credible evidence', but not Vitamin C: 'nothing credible there'. What about fish oils? 'Oh, well, they're probably a good thing – I don't take them, but I do eat fish.' He also exercises every other day, although he regrets that he has had to give up golf for lack of time.

Guarente is a humble pioneer. 'My goal was not to make yeast and mice live longer,' he says, his long, white hands flapping expressively, 'but to understand what limits them. I didn't think we would get to humans.' He doesn't want to abolish ageing – indeed, he doesn't think it's possible – but he does 'want to add life to our years'. And he's not alone. Other researchers are thinking along similar lines.

Unleashing the Restorers to Challenge the Wreckers in Our Bodies

While Leonard Guarente was studying yeast in Boston, in 1993, the biologist Cynthia Kenyon was peering through her microscope at tiny roundworms at the University of California, San Francisco. The way Kenyon talks about these worms – named c-elegans – you get the impression she became rather fond of them. They live for only 30 days, and Kenyon describes the 'tragic arc of that life' wiggling vibrantly for the first 15 days, then slowing down as their tissues deteriorated. Their last ten days would be spent waving their heads feebly, barely able to move.

To their own surprise, Kenyon and her team made an astonishing discovery. By partially disabling a single gene – called daf-2 – they found they could double the worms' lifespan.[7]

Kenyon describes looking up from the normal worms, which were dying, to the ones in the culture dish, still acting young at the same age. 'It was a creepy feeling, my hair stood up,' she tells me, in her soft Californian lilt. 'Like we had done something you weren't really supposed to do. You think, oh my, they should be dead. We made our worms live longer.'

The mutant worms kept wiggling around, almost until death. They didn't have a prolonged doddery stage like the normal worms. This was revolutionary, a glimpse of God. Kenyon had identified another gene which could be manipulated to dramatically slow ageing.

These findings apply to humans too. A study of Ashkenazy Jews living in New York City found that those who made it to 90 or 100 were more likely to have the daf-2 gene mutation. 'It doesn't mean someone at 90 can run a marathon,' Kenyon says, 'but they're ageing more slowly and they look younger. They *are* younger.'

Do Our Bodies Just Wear Out?

It is widely believed that we age because the DNA in our cells becomes progressively damaged – by radiation, pollution and stress, and by the natural process of cell division. Most of our cells turn over regularly: our skin cells renew around every 20 days, our bones about every three years, and DNA damage is occurring all the time. There are about 10,000 breaks in DNA every day, in every cell.[8]

When we are young, our bodies are amazingly good at repairing these breaks, through the churning molecular biology of our cells. But this repair process consumes huge amounts of energy, and it weakens as we get older. More breaks can persist in cells like heart cells, which never divide or divide rarely. All this damage is cumulative. As a result, we become less and less resistant to disease. That's why cancer, stroke and cardiovascular disease – the three leading causes of death in developed countries – mostly hit older people, not the young. Visit an intensive care unit at any hospital and most of the patients will have something in common: they're old.

An important aspect of this decline, according to some biogerontologists, is our metabolism. The repair processes use a lot of oxygen, but oxygen is not always fully metabolised. This unleashes 'free radicals', atoms with unpaired electrons, which whizz around causing mischief, stealing electrons from other molecules. While these are mostly mopped up by antioxidant molecules in the body, some get missed so changes to our genes gradually accumulate, causing damage like rust getting at a car. Many people take antioxidant supplements to ward off the effects of free radicals, but even proponents of the theory (and the free radical theory is not universally accepted) say there is little evidence that antioxidant supplements work.

In summary, ageing seems to weaken the restorers – the good proteins and genes like the sirtuins – which help with cell repair. These restorers no longer stand up to the body's biological wreckers, like the daf-2 gene. By weakening the daf-2 gene's activity, Kenyon's team allowed the cell restorers to work better. The cells seemed to think they were younger – so behaved as if they were.

Can We Live Forever?

The oldest-known human, the Frenchwoman Jeanne Calment, lived to the age of 122.[9] Having outlived both her daughter and her grandson in Arles, France, she had no one to bequeath her apartment to. She sold it to a lawyer in return for a monthly sum to be paid until her death. By the time she died, in 1997, the monthly payments amounted to twice the value of the property.

There is no special explanation for why Calment lived so long. And no one has beaten her record. Many scientists think that around 120 probably represents an outer biological age limit for humankind. There are many more centenarians than there used to be. But there has been – as yet – no paradigm shift.

That might have something to do with the number of times our cells can divide. In 1961, Leonard Hayflick, Professor of Anatomy at the University of California, discovered that normal human cells only replicate a certain number of times before they die. Hayflick and his assistant put the cells in dishes in his laboratory and watched them reproduce by making copies of themselves. At first, the cells replicated so rapidly and 'luxuriantly', as Hayflick later described it, that they could not save them all. But after a while – when the longest-lasting cells had divided about 50 times – everything ground to a halt. The cells stopped dividing.

Hayflick called this state 'senescence' – the period before death when cells are still alive, but have lost the ability to divide. That point, when cells start to die, is known as the Hayflick Limit and is thought to apply to every living creature.

We don't just suddenly hit the Hayflick Limit and keel over. Our tissues age once too many cells become senescent; our wounds take longer to heal and we are more susceptible to infections. The senescent cells sit around, feebly calling on immune cells for help, causing inflammation. This can lead to a prolonged and miserable period of senescence at the end of life.

Hayflick discovered that cells have an internal stopwatch, which tracks the number of cell divisions.[10] This stopwatch is linked to tiny protective caps, called telomeres, on the ends of each chromosome. Every time a cell divides, the telomeres shorten and fray, rather like the plastic coating on the end of a shoelace. When telomeres get too short, the cell ceases to divide and the mitochondria which produce energy in those cells fade away. Telomeres are by no means the only cause of senescence – and I don't recommend that you necessarily rush off and get your telomeres tested for an exorbitant sum. Mice have lived longer when given telomerase, an enzyme which rebuilds the telomeres. But no one has yet found a way to give human beings more telomerase without fuelling cancer – because unlimited cell division leads to tumours.[11]

The 'Biologically Immortal' Creatures

Telomerase is an example of an enzyme which is beneficial to us in early life, but can turn deadly later. The hormone testosterone is similar: it makes young men stronger, but exposes older men to a higher risk of prostate cancer.

When you study ageing, you begin to see these evolutionary trade-offs everywhere. It brings the whole subject into focus. The daf-2 gene, it turns out, is essential in early life. Embryos can't develop without it. But when it expresses itself later on, as Cynthia Kenyon saw with her worms, it's a wrecker.

Scientists who are trying to extend life are battling a fundamental evolutionary trade-off between longevity and reproduction. Evolutionary theory would suggest that we have fulfilled our purpose once we have passed our reproductive years, improved and sustained the gene pool, and perhaps cared for grandchildren. Animals which survive through a famine on restricted calories often become infertile during that period, investing their slender resources into survival. And some living creatures don't age like humans do.

In 2007, an unsuspecting fisherman in Maine got a shock when he hauled in a lobster with giant claws, which was estimated from its weight to be 180 years old. Lobsters are 'biologically immortal'. They keep on growing unless they are caught or injured, and they become more fertile as they age, because as they grow bigger, they are less likely to become prey. They evolved to have fewer genes that are beneficial earlier but detrimental later.

Lobsters don't actually live for ever: they grow by moulting their shells and when the shell gets too big, they run out of energy to moult. Then they die quickly, rather as an old person might die of pneumonia. They don't get cancer, despite having high levels of telomerase, because they possess other genes that mediate telomerase differently to humans. And they remain fertile – as do some other creatures, including Blanding's turtles.

Super-Centenarians Have Less Chance of Dying

Although no one has yet outlived Jeanne Calment, a strange phenomenon has been observed in very old humans: our chances of dying start to level off if we can make it to 105.

A team led by the Italian demographer Elisabetta Barbi looked at records for the 3,800 Italians aged over 105, mostly women, who were alive between 2009 and 2015.[12] Up to the age of 80, the team found that death rates increased exponentially. Beyond that point they slowed down, approaching a 'plateau' after the age of 105. At 105, your risk of dying is 50 per cent – admittedly high – but beyond that age, it never seems to get any higher. We are as likely to cheat death aged 110, or 115, as we are at 105. And when we do die, we are likely to die quickly, of organ failure, rather than from any prolonged chronic disease. That sounds quite attractive – although being 105 is not a breeze.

Another study, of 'super-centenarians' over 110, reinforces the view that very old people may evade prolonged senescence.[13] Almost half were still functionally independent. Few had diabetes or Parkinson's disease, and they were virtually immune to vascular diseases.

It seems that very old humans may defy the Gompertz Law, a mathematical rule which says that the risk of dying rises exponentially with age. Defined in 1825 by the British mathematician Benjamin Gompertz, this law states that humans' risk of dying roughly doubles every eight years after the age of 30. But Barbi's findings suggest this may cease to be true after 105.

One other creature defies the Gompertz Law: the naked mole rat. This hideously ugly pink rodent, found in the arid deserts of East Africa, has the same risk of dying whether it is three years old, or 30.[14] It is the longest-lived rodent on the planet, and highly resistant to cancer. According to 2018 research carried out at Calico, Google's anti-ageing spin-off in San Francisco, it does not grow old like any other creature.

Naked mole rats possess what is known as 'negligible senescence'. We don't know why, although this has given rise to a great many theories. The bearded gerontologist Dr Aubrey de Grey, who founded the SENS (Strategies for Engineered Negligible Senescence) Research Foundation to research routes to immortality, believes naked mole rats repair their cells' damage as it occurs. De Grey famously said that he believes there is already someone alive today – maybe someone aged 50 or 60 – who will live to be 1,000. He founded the Methuselah Mouse Prize, in 2003, for any researcher who could stretch the lifespan of a mouse to unprecedented lengths.

De Grey is a controversial figure. Two years after the Methuselah Mouse Prize was established, Jason Pontin, editor of the respected *MIT Technology Review*, offered a $20,000 prize to any molecular biologist who could demonstrate that de Grey's Strategies for Engineered Negligible Senescence were fantasy. None of the applicants was judged to have absolutely disproved SENS. The entrepreneur and investor Jim Mellon says that 'some of Aubrey's prophecies are slowly wending their way into the realms of reality'.[15] But Pontin still believes, as do many scientists, that de Grey's desire to re-engineer the nucleus of a cell is impossible with any technology we can currently foresee.

The Compounds Which Could be Elixirs of Youth

'There is no maximum human lifespan,' proclaims David Sinclair, the softly spoken Australian who is Professor of Genetics at Harvard Medical School. 'Yes,' he shrugs, 'if you look back in history, there is an apparent lifespan of about 120. But that's like saying in 1900 that humans will never achieve powered flight.' To make his point, grinning, he pushes a large photograph of the Wright brothers towards me across the table. There they are, in black and white, the inventors of the world's first successful aeroplane.

A little unnerved, I take a breath. We are sitting in Sinclair's office, surrounded by neatly stacked books, but his personality seems bigger than the room. Although we have already talked at length on the phone, I didn't realise how intense he would be in person. Wiry, elfin-looking, he's wearing a dark grey T-shirt with 'Totally Weird' written on it. He speaks quietly, but makes big statements: he projects a powerful charisma.

David Sinclair is a wunderkind. Just 48, he has already founded nine biotech companies, been an inventor on 35 patents, and been named one of the 100 Most Influential People in the World by *Time* magazine. He has been published in peer-reviewed journals all over the world. Citations and framed magazine articles adorn the walls. Sinclair does not speak with the careful restraint of most scientists I meet: he comes across as ebullient, almost mischievously optimistic.

Sinclair started his career working for Leonard Guarente, and his work has partly been inspired by the discoveries of sirtuins that he was involved in at Guarente's lab. Since then he has been an ardent proponent of many compounds, some of which have been investigated by pharmaceutical companies.

One of the earliest compounds Sinclair backed was resveratrol, an antioxidant found in red wine, which is thought to be a powerful sirtuin activator.[16] Mice given resveratrol have lived substantially longer than their peers. A human would need to drink hundreds of glasses of wine to get the same effect, however, and no one has yet proved conclusively that it is safe to be taken in high doses – although Sinclair argues that mice have consumed it in large doses and become sleek and athletic.

There is some scepticism in the field about resveratrol. In 2010, the company GlaxoSmithKline plc ended its clinical trials of a proprietary formulation of resveratrol, which it had bought through its acquisition of Sirtris Pharmaceuticals, a company founded by Sinclair. There are concerns about side effects.[17] It's notable, however, how many Americans I have met (all men, as it happens), who are buying resveratrol from health food stores. 'In ten years, it'll be much clearer which of these things are miracles and which are duds,' one told me recently. 'But I could be dead by then.'

Undeterred, Sinclair's lab is looking at a number of other molecules which could slow ageing. One is Metformin, a prescription drug derived from French lilac, which is widely used for diabetic patients because it increases sensitivity to the hormone insulin and lowers blood-sugar levels. But Metformin has other, unexpected powers: it seems to slow the growth of some cancers. A 2014 study at Cardiff University found that type 2 diabetics who were given Metformin lived longer than non-diabetics who were not on the drug.[18] This is a simply extraordinary finding, with potentially huge implications: not only for diabetics, but for everyone. Because as we age, our organs become more resistant to insulin.

Metformin is now the lead compound in a clinical trial to attempt to slow ageing.[19] Led by Dr Nir Barzilai, founder of the US Institute for Aging Research, the trial aims to test whether age-related diseases can be delayed in a group of non-diabetic older people who take the drug, compared with a control group who don't. Barzilai's aim is to convince regulators to approve ageing as a specific condition. If they do, ageing itself could become a target for future medications.

Human trials are vital, because – to state the obvious – rodents are not the same as people. One Taiwanese study suggested that diabetics who have taken Metformin for more than 12 years may be at greater risk of Parkinson's and Alzheimer's.[20] However, I've met longevity experts who say they are taking Metformin, buying it online with no prescription.

One of Sinclair's most recent discoveries concerns a compound found in broccoli and cabbage. NMN (nicotinamide mononucleotide) seems to mimic the effects of calorie restriction, because the body converts it into the wonder molecule NAD.

Sinclair becomes hugely animated, talking about his team's recent experiments treating mice with NMN.[21] They found that signs of ageing in the tissue and muscles of the older mice reversed to the point where they could no longer tell the difference between a two-year-old mouse and a four-month-old one. 'The cells of the old mice were indistinguishable from the young,' he says excitedly, tossing me a copy of the journal *Cell*, in which the findings have been published. 'The mice are leaner, they have more energy, they can run further on the treadmill.'

Human trials are to begin soon: if they go well, Sinclair thinks a safe drug could come to market in between three and five years. He claims NMN is already pretty safe to take, because it's 'a supplement, like a larger version of Vitamin B3. We are simply replenishing what's been lost.' He himself has been taking NMN and says he feels less tired, although he agrees this is not robust evidence.

Why is he so confident about these compounds, NMN, resveratrol and Metformin? It turns out that Sinclair's longest-running human experiment is his own father. Mr Sinclair senior has been taking some of these molecules for over a decade. 'My father escaped the Hungarian Revolution in '56 and went to Australia,' he confides. 'He wasn't expecting a long life; his mother spent the last ten years in a nursing home. We have what you might call terrible genes. He retired at 67 and thought he'd travel for a few years. He started on resveratrol 12 years ago. He didn't admit to believing in the research, but he said, "What have I got to lose?"'

Sinclair reaches to his right, over to the desk. He picks up a framed photograph of three smiling, energetic-looking hikers on a hillside. One, looking youthful, is his dad. 'Eighteen months ago,' he says slowly, 'he started taking NMN. It's remarkable to see what has happened. He is 78, all his peers are dead or can barely walk around the block, but he feels younger than he did in his thirties. He goes hiking and white-water rafting. He doesn't get tired, he goes to the gym and he is the fittest in his group.'

Sinclair says he has been taking resveratrol for ten years himself, and that other members of his family are taking some of these molecules too. Other scientists are less convinced. They point out that some diabetics have stopped taking Metformin because it causes stomach upsets and diarrhoea; and that Glaxo ended its 2010 trial. They fear Sinclair is over-hyping compounds whose effects can only ever be limited. But Sinclair is bullish. He says that his own body age has fallen in the past two years, according to information he gets from a firm called Inside Tracker. (He sits on the board of this firm, which uses AI to analyse genetic data.) And, he believes, these compounds are only the start. Sinclair has become fascinated by the epigenome, the system in our bodies which controls which genes are active at any given moment. When we are young, this system works efficiently, with chemical signals firing and keeping the 'wreckers' at bay. As we get older, he says, these signals become confused, by epigenetic 'noise', which eventually leads to senescence. Sun damage and radiation, Sinclair says, are both causes of epigenetic noise. He won't go through airport scanners for that reason. When he tells them what he does for a living, the airport staff let him go round the side, he tells me. Since hearing this story, I have started to wonder whether I, too, should avoid the scanners – though I've so far felt too embarrassed to ask.

Sinclair's lab is working to decode some of the epigenetic pathways through which restorers and wreckers operate. Resveratrol and Metformin trigger epigenetic pathways, which promote sirtuins.

The First Human Ageing Trial

In 2014, in what has been called 'the first human ageing trial', hundreds of Australians and New Zealanders over 65 were given a drug derived from a bacterium found in the soil on Easter Island in the South Pacific. 'Rapamycin' is named after 'Rapa Nui', the native word for Easter Island. Used by doctors for years, as an immunosuppressant, to prevent organ transplant rejection, it has also been shown to extend the lifespan of mice by 20 per cent.[22]

Researchers gave a derivative of rapamycin to patients who were about to get a flu vaccine. They found that the patients' immune systems responded more effectively than their peers: as if they were younger.[23] This was a very important finding: it looks as though rapamycin may slow down the decline of the immune system as we age. It works by suppressing something called the mTOR complex,[24] a set of genes which regulate metabolism. Inhibiting mTOR achieves a similar effect to calorie restriction, pushing cells into survival mode and extending life.

This process has made mTOR an important target for ageing research. The hunt is on for ways to gently inhibit mTOR, without creating side effects. A study is even under way in Seattle, to see if rapamycin can extend the lifespan of middle-aged dogs.

Using Stem Cells to Regenerate Bodies

There has been a great deal of discussion about the prospect of using stem cells to manufacture new organs as our bodies wear out. Some of these, 'pluripotent' stem cells, can be used to make any other kind of cell in the body. They have already been used to fix age-related macular degeneration in people with failing eyesight,[25] and to treat spinal cord injuries. If we could engineer more of them, we might be able to reset the clock of ageing – by using them to grow a new kidney, for example, with none of the usual worries about whether the body will reject the transplant – because the body has grown the organ itself.

Zebrafish already do this: they can regrow their own heart tissue. Scientists at King's College London have found parallels between the way that zebrafish regenerate hearts, and the way adult cells repair damaged skin. Moreover, we can now avoid the ethical dilemma of harvesting embryos, because the Japanese scientist Shinya Yamanaka has proved that mature adult cells can be reprogrammed to become pluripotent.[26]

We are probably at least ten years away from being able to safely regenerate any organ. Few stem-cell therapies have been through clinical trials and there are growing concerns about the number of dubious clinics[27] proliferating around the world, with reports that some patients have been blinded by clinics claiming to be able to improve sight. This is always the danger when science moves faster than regulators. But scientists like David Sinclair argue that regulators need to take a wholly different approach to ageing.

Should We Treat Ageing as a Disease?

The discoveries I have outlined in this chapter suggest that ageing may be a syndrome which is partially treatable, not simply the inevitable accumulation of defects over time. Many bio-gerontologists now think that ageing itself should be categorised as a disease.

Conventional medicine treats one disease at a time: cancer, or heart disease, or stroke. But even if we manage to eliminate one, that would bring us only an extra four or five years of life,[28] because something else will get us instead. Plummeting rates of death from heart attack, while a great success, offer up more future victims to dementia. Same with cancer. That's because the major driver of these diseases is ageing. We used to think that ageing was not a variable we could modify. But we must, if we are to significantly increase the healthspan.

Sinclair, Kenyon, Guarente and their colleagues offer the possibility that we could target the biology which underlies ageing itself. By triggering the ancient genetic circuits which protect cells and tissues in response to stresses like famine, they have been able to rejuvenate whole organisms. Anti-ageing drugs which sparked those circuits could therefore slow the progress of several diseases, not just one.[29] Yet most research funding is still directed towards individual diseases, rather than at ageing itself. Sinclair claims that ageing research receives about one hundredth the investment that is given to heart disease and diabetes.

'The medical establishment is in denial,' says David Sinclair. 'They think that what I'm trying to do is impossible or trite. But the tragedy of twenty-first century medicine is that it only addresses one disease at a time. The approach the ageing research community is taking is to say let's not keep one aspect of the body alive, not just one organ or tissue, but let's harness the body's natural defences against decay and disease and keep all the organs healthy and young and resilient so that, yes, you can take a drug for your diabetes, but you won't get cancer as a side effect, and you'll be able to climb mountains like my father does at 78.'

When ageing is thought to be immutable, it creates an unusual hurdle for scientists trying to bring anti-ageing drugs to market. Regulators will only license drugs which target defined diseases. Ageing itself is not defined as a disease, because regulators do not think of ageing as something which is treatable, let alone curable. However this makes it difficult to persuade pharmaceutical companies to invest, as they may not get a licence to sell their inventions.

Every 20 years, the World Health Organization updates the way it categorises disease. A huge lobbying process is now under way to try and convince it to include ageing as a specific condition. However campaigners fighting for research funds for cancer or Alzheimer's worry that precious funds could be diverted into a wild goose chase. Scepticism is not helped by the profusion of snake-oil salesmen in the anti-ageing space, peddling dubious treatments. Moreover, improving people's chances of a healthy old age seems more legitimate and worthy than seeking an elusive elixir of immortality. As Bill Gates has said, 'It seems pretty egocentric, while we still have malaria and TB, for rich people to fund things so they can live longer.'[30]

The potential benefits of drugs which could prolong healthy lifespan are enormous. If ageing were defined as a disease, this could unlock serious investment from the pharmaceutical industry. It might also change the way we think. We start to fear old age long before we enter it. Improving our chances of living better for longer could be hugely liberating. What's at stake could be nothing less than a revolution in how we experience our final decades.

The New Masters of the Universe

In the course of writing this book, I have come across a surprising number of people who are taking many of the compounds I've mentioned in this chapter. They are members of an exclusive club: rich, educated people who have read the research and decided to take a risk. Talking to some of them, I can't help thinking that getting ahead of ageing is, perhaps, the ultimate status symbol.

If these drugs are comprehensively proven to work, it is vital that they do not remain the preserve of the rich. David Sinclair has pledged, if he succeeds in producing anti-ageing medicines approved by the FDA, that he will make them widely available, and 'not just developed countries, because I think this is just too important to provide the drugs to people who can afford them and leave out large sections of the globe'. That is a laudable ambition.

Anti-ageing drugs could be as important and transformational in the twenty-first century as antibiotics were in the twentieth. And the companies which will dominate that space will be some of the largest in the world – perhaps the rivals to Google and Amazon. Watch this space.

7

Out of the Ghetto

Everyone needs a neighbourhood

WHICH OF THESE TWO statements do you agree with more?

'Generally speaking, most people can be trusted'; or:

'Generally speaking, you can't be too careful in dealing with people'.

When this question was put to residents of 14 different European countries,[1] the trusting people who agreed with the first statement reported being in much better health than those who tended to be suspicious. The researchers, from the World Health Organization, found the most positive attitudes, and best health, in places with high 'social capital': trust between neighbours, repeat interactions and helpful actions reciprocated.

'The key to healthy ageing is relationships, relationships, relationships,' wrote George Vaillant, the psychiatrist who led the Harvard Study of Adult Development. This 80-year study tracked a group of Harvard undergraduates, and some poorer citizens from the other end of town, for their entire lives. Some became factory workers, others lawyers. Some became addicts, others suffered mental illness. Some made it from the Boston slums to the pinnacle of society; others made the journey in the opposite direction. But wherever they landed up, the ones with strong social connections were happier, lived longer and were physically healthier than the ones who felt isolated.

'When the study began, nobody cared about empathy or attachment,' Vaillant said. But happy marriages and strong friendships turned out to be vital. It wasn't the number of relationships which mattered, he found, but their quality. People who felt they had relationships they could rely on had sharper brains at 80 and reported being happier, even on days when they were in physical pain.

There's probably no better buffer for stress than the security of feeling we have friends to rely on. That's what Okinawans have, through their *moai* group (see page 3), and it's what all of us need. As children move away to pursue careers, and spouses and friends die, too many of us are left isolated, without people who are geographically close enough to rely on. A lack of social connections is said to be as damaging to our health as smoking 15 cigarettes a day.[2]

My father was extremely lucky in this regard. Fifteen years before he died, he was living around the corner from me in London, but he felt oppressed by his upstairs neighbours, who were noisy, so he upped sticks and moved into a part of London which feels like a village, with small houses and narrow streets. He already had one friend there and rapidly made many more, all considerably younger than him. One of his neighbours saved his life, by rushing round to his house after realising he hadn't seen him in the street (he let himself in with the spare key and found my father trapped in his bath). At his funeral, which was held in the local church before we all repaired to the local pub, people I'd never even heard of turned up. It was like an old-fashioned country village, right in the middle of one of the world's largest capital cities. It was a true neighbourhood.

Re-Creating the Neighbourhood

In times gone past, the neighbourhood was somewhere you could feel safe. Where people looked out for each other and would notice if things were not right. It might be oppressive at times – Victorian novels are full of gossipy spinsters twitching curtains – but not as lonely as our modern world. The rise of anonymous city living, the fragmentation of families and the decline of organised religion have removed natural meeting places, and segregated the generations. Loneliness and anxiety are bad for our health.[3] They can even, one study suggested, predict dementia.

There is a huge hunger to re-create community. You can see it everywhere. But people aren't sure how to do it. You can't force them to join clubs. Humans are proud creatures: few of us readily admit to being lonely.

So, how do we do it?

The Dutch academic Lillian Linders has written about what she calls the 'request scruple' – our reluctance to seek help because we fear dependency, or we idealise autonomy. Studying a relatively poor, industrial part of Holland, she found that residents were often prepared to help others in principle. In practice they were wary of actually offering: Linders defined this as the 'support scruple'. But they would help if others overcame their reluctance to ask, and they were far more likely to do so if they lived in close promixity.

Many years ago I visited Southwark Circle, set up in a part of south London to help isolated people over 50 offer services to each other. I met an old guy taking language lessons from a Spanish lady, both laughing about his hopelessness in learning vocabulary. But the Spanish wasn't really the point. An evaluation of Southwark Circle found that it had reduced the number of 'non-essential' visits to GPs, because lonely people were instead forging new friendships. Membership organisations like this help overcome our natural scruples – because they are based on reciprocal exchange.

In Beacon Hill, Boston, Massachusetts, one group of middle-aged people realised 20 years ago that they already lived in a functioning neighbourhood. If they could deepen ties between residents, they thought, they might be able to see out their days in their own homes, looking out for themselves and for each other. They created a membership organisation called Beacon Hill Village, which has now spawned more than 350 other 'villages' around the world.

Beacon Hill Village

In Joy Street, Boston, Susan McWhinney Morse, 84, recounts the evening in 1999 when she and ten local residents got together to figure out a way to avoid the kind of old age they watched their parents endure.

'We all talked about our experiences with our parents,' Susan tells me. 'About our dismay at the way nursing homes were isolating and vandalising. We felt we knew better what was needed than the social work agencies. And we wanted to keep our minds and bodies going.'

The group who met that evening were aged between 55 and 80: some were retired, others still working. They decided to create a club which would put on social events, organise exercise classes to keep fit, do weekly grocery shopping trips and offer lifts to medical appointments.

And so was born Beacon Hill Village – amid the historic ivy-covered rowhouses and old-fashioned lantern streetlights which draw the tourists walking up to the Massachusetts State House to join the Freedom Trail. It's a chilly day. I've walked up from the Red Line subway at Charles and the steep red brick sidewalks are slippery. The hills are famously vertiginous, almost as steep as San Francisco, and I observe that the cobbles must be murder in winter, but Susan, leaning on a stick, says cheerfully that it's her 'aerobic exercise': 'They say folks in New York are healthier because they have to climb up and down all those steps to the subway. It's the same here. I'm surrounded by people with new hips, and I live in a duplex.'

Wearing a red tunic over a black silk shirt, with a full head of white hair and sharp eyes behind her black framed glasses, Susan McWhinney Morse has a commanding presence. She became convinced of the need to keep people in their own homes, she says, after visiting her mother-in-law in a care home: 'It was awful. We used to take her out for picnics so she didn't have to sit in the dreadful dining room. One Saturday, we were told she was downstairs with the others. When we got down she was in the doorway in her wheelchair, feet firmly on the floor. The nurse said, "She's being difficult, she won't let us push her." But that was the only way she could say "no": to put her feet on the floor.'

The group which founded the Village laid out clear principles of self-reliance and voluntary co-operation, very much in keeping with Boston's Puritan, seventeenth-century roots. The Village must be driven and funded by the members, not by the state. It should be open to everyone – a fund has been raised quietly to help the less prosperous afford the membership fee. And it keeps its overheads low: 'We were determined we would never own property or have a large staff,' says Susan. The offices are tiny, and sparse. When I visit, a fierce debate is raging about whether to lease a van.

The desire to remain independent has been a powerful motivator. When I ask Susan whether she would ever move in with her children, she looks appalled. 'I spent 20 years getting them to be independent. They work full-time, they have children of their own, and complicated lives. I'd rather have lunch with my daughter than have her take me to a colonoscopy. Plus, I want to eat and sleep and work and walk on *my* schedule, not anyone else's.'

Even with such determined leaders, creating the network was not all plain sailing. 'The first night, 60 people signed up,' says Susan. 'We were delighted. But the next month, we only got one new member.' The mistake was that they were calling themselves a 'virtual retirement community', which sounded like something for has-beens. 'No one liked it. They'd say, "I will join when I'm older, when I'm ready." We did not understand the ageism of our own population.'

They changed the name and now there is a plethora of heart-warming stories about neighbours' generosity. One much-loved member called Tina joined the Village when she retired from nursing. She had never married, had worked incredibly hard and knew few people, so she threw herself into Village life. Her 90th birthday party in the Village is said to have been 'a great bash'. But two years later, Tina fell over, broke her femur and was taken to hospital. The doctor told her she needed to go into a nursing home.

'Tina said no, she was going home,' explains Laura Connors, CEO of Beacon Hill Village and one of the few paid members of staff. 'But it was four steps up from the street to her front door, then you had to push a heavy door and get into the elevator.' Tina finally made it, with the help of a friend, but when she got into her bedroom she found the bed was too high, so she called the Village. 'Within minutes,' says Laura, 'there were two sets of neighbours at her door. One couple took Tina's mattress off the bed, put it on the floor and helped her get into it. Another played games with Tina to pass the time, while the fourth neighbour made some calls and eventually managed to find Tina a new apartment.'

That's the kind of support we would all like to be able to draw on in times of need. The kind which comes from friendship and mutual respect. Susan emphasises that the Village is not a social work organisation but a voluntary network. She had to keep explaining this, she says, when she started being invited around the country to give talks. 'I would get asked things like: "How do you know your clients (a word we never use) are taking their meds?" Or: "How can you keep them from falling?" I would say that we know these things are important, but that we try to help people be responsible for themselves.'

The Village co-ordinates resources. It will make referrals to home helps, for example, but not provide them. 'You can call the Village and ask: how do I get a plumber? Or how do I get social security?' says Laura. 'There's a real voice here, it's not "dial 1 for a plumber, 2 for social security", but it's a person, often a volunteer, who listens to you and responds.'

Murray Frank, a former lecturer, joined the Village after his wife died. 'I had a very good marriage, it left a huge hole. Someone dragged me to a meeting. Basically, you go to a meeting and ask a question and pretty soon you're on the committee!' he grins. Then, earnestly: 'For quite a while I wouldn't go out on my own. The only interesting thing I did was go to a concert with fellow members.'

Dapper in a tweed jacket, with a neatly trimmed beard and twinkling eyes, Murray claims to be 91. I am genuinely amazed. 'You don't know what someone of 91 is supposed to look like!' he chuckles, pleased. He now enjoys going on trips and meeting people. Last week he went on a trip around the public library and met ten neighbours he'd never seen before.

At his age, Murray says that he often feels invisible. 'You walk up to a department store counter,' he drawls in his strong Boston accent, 'and there's me and a young person. See who the clerk serves first!' He rolls his eyes. Nevertheless, he doesn't want to be stuck with the superannuated. 'I don't want a retirement home,' he says. 'All they are is old people and misery. Here, where I live, I'm surrounded by children and adults working. And when I need it, I have the Village.'

These people did not wait for government agencies to decide how they were going to age. They got on and created a stronger community, one which means retirement does not have to be lonely, or unoccupied. While Beacon Hill is a prosperous area, variants on its model have been replicated in far less well-off places. At its heart is something money can't buy: a core of determined people acting together. Susan says fondly that Murray is a 'stalwart'. He calls her, joshingly, the 'Mother Superior'.

'We have been extraordinarily lucky,' Susan reflects. 'But I believe passionately that groups of people can move mountains.'

The Retirement Village

Many people still dream of retiring to the coast and tending their garden. But rather than retreat at that time of life, they actually need to build wider networks for what may turn out to be a longer future than they imagine. In Australia and the US, one answer has been to build 'retirement villages', where couples can whizz around on golf carts, attend yoga classes and even woo a new sweetheart, if a spouse dies. Its success is shown in the numbers: ten times as many Australians live in such purpose-built retirement communities as Brits: 5.7 per cent of the over-65 population.[4] In Australia this is a particularly popular option for those who want easy access to medical help and facilities, and for those who worry about their health: over 70 per cent of residents have used an emergency call button in their facilities. Australian villages tend to be near existing communities: over half of village residents move less than 10 kilometres from their house.[5]

Swathes of these villages are now being built in China, with names like 'Golden Heights', or 'Golden Sunshine', channelling the original 'Sun City' retirement community in Florida. Some are backed by insurance companies. One such home, on the eastern outskirts of Beijing, has been built around a hospital to provide added reassurance. In Europe a scaled-down version is often called 'sheltered housing', with self-contained flats around a communal area and a 24-hour warden.

Some of these developments are well designed. They bring comfort to many people who have the cash and don't want to burden their adult children. But they are expensive, so will only ever cater for a few. Those which are located far from cities can be incompatible with any desire to unretire. And many have struggled to create a deep sense of community. That's partly because they often insist that everyone must be over 65, skewing the community to something a little artificial. But it's also because their residents have mostly bought into the facilities, not into any uniting philosophy.

A different approach was pioneered in Denmark and the Netherlands in the 1960s. Groups of individuals banded together in 'co-housing' developments with self-contained flats, communal living spaces and a philosophy of active mutual support. The natural descendants of the 1920s New York co-op apartments, these are often more natural communities, because the residents come together in pursuit of a particular way of living. Unlike retirement villages, which are run by developers in pursuit of profit, co-housing developments are run by the residents themselves, with shared values they believe in.

Sisters Are Doing It for Themselves

'Being part of running this place makes me feel so positive about life,' says Angela Ratcliffe, 85, who lives in New Ground, the UK's first co-housing development for older people. 'I think the most important thing about ageing is keeping control. No one's said "you need looking after" – it keeps us active.'

Angela lives in the New Ground complex in north London, with a group of other women aged between 51 and 89. Her apartment is one of 25 in this light and airy development, set around a flourishing garden which the residents tend themselves, in a quiet Victorian terraced street near the Underground. It has taken, incredibly, 18 years of campaigning to build this complex, which opened in 2016. Some of the original campaigners died before they ever got to see it.

The spaces are designed to help casual interaction. The kitchen windows look out onto a walkway and the corridors take people past the common room. 'You can wave if there's someone in there,' says Angela, 'you can pop in for a chat. But you don't have to. We all lead our own lives. You can be in your own flat, looking out on a lovely garden, seeing other people and you don't have to be involved with them if you don't want to – but if you do, they're there.'

Like many of her New Ground neighbours, Angela is divorced. She started out as an actress, became a marriage guidance counsellor (she smiles at the irony), learned to cook for her husband and daughter, then later became a probation officer and a child and family therapist. When I ask why there are no men in the group, I don't know whether to expect an ideological rant. But she simply says, mildly, that 'the generation of women who started trying to get this going had left partners who thought it was their role to run things. I imagine it will be different for the next generation.' Whatever the individual reasons, this is clearly a liberation for many of these women.

The origins of New Ground are quite similar to those of Beacon Hill Village: a desire to remain independent and not 'be done to'. In 1998, a group of six women who already knew each other became aware that they were feeling less safe in the city as they grew older and didn't want to become isolated. Scattered across London, they decided to create the UK's first co-housing community for older women.

The members of this Older Women's Co-Housing (OWCH) group are all very different, but they share a set of common, carefully established principles. These include sharing responsibility, supporting each other, combating ageist stereotypes, caring for the environment and being part of the wider community. This is not a gated community, a group in retreat from the world. On the contrary, it wants to embrace it.

Maria Brenton, aged 73, one of the early members, had studied the Dutch approach to keeping people happy and active in older age. 'They share their old age together,' she says. 'It gives them a conviviality.' She believes that co-housing can reduce strain on the health and social care system[6] by keeping people healthier for longer – indeed, that was an explicit aim of the founders. Local councils, however, disagreed. They feared that bringing more older women into the borough would increase demands on the social care budget.

The project turned out to be a long exercise in tenacity. The group had considerable trouble finding a developer or council who would partner with them, partly because they were determined to include some tenants who couldn't afford to buy their own flats in the development and were on state benefits. At New Ground, 17 flats are owned by their occupants; eight are for social renters on assured tenancies. Developers didn't like the mix of leasehold and social housing. Councils wanted to choose which social housing tenants got a place in the development – something which would have completely undermined the group's need to pick people who shared their philosophy.

Maria describes the hostility she encountered from local authorities. 'They'd say to me: "How can you justify looking for public funds and letting people choose their own neighbours?"' she explains. 'But I'd say: "Your monocultural estates haven't worked too well, have they?"' The Netherlands, she would point out, encourages mixed tenure communities.

After 13 years of meeting, discussing, looking for sites, losing sites, marketing, lobbying and despairing, the Hanover Housing Association stepped in and bought the site. The women were able to choose the architects and worked with them to design the new building. It's clear that the whole process has been tremendously bonding, although OWCH stresses that it's ultimately the people who make the community, not the houses. There's little point in striving for a lovely building if the occupants don't gel.

It is striking that none of the women have yet needed to turn to nursing care. 'People have had minor crises,' Angela tells me. 'We have prepared meals if someone's ill, or fetched and carried and taken them to hospital – it's what you'd do for any neighbours who are friends, if you knew they needed help.' Living here, someone in need is quickly spotted – if their blinds are drawn, or if they haven't been seen. No one fears that they could lie for days without anyone noticing.

Building the Future

Given the demonstrable benefits, it's surprising that there are not more projects like New Ground. There are about 300 co-housing developments in the Netherlands, and around 160 in the US – some for older people. But developers remain more interested in constructing 'retirement villages' for the well-off, or grim, one-bed apartments for poorer pensioners, which have no space for a grandchild, or a lifetime's paraphernalia. There's not much else available.

In the UK, a third of over-65s now live on their own. Two-thirds are women.[7] But many councils resist older people's housing, fearing the resulting burden on public services. And good sites are expensive, making it hard to build affordable developments with communal space. Yet if we could build better housing for older people, we could free up much-needed space for younger ones.

'We need to shuffle the pack and get younger people into the larger homes, and older people into lovely, purpose-built accommodation without stairs,' says Lord Richard Best, social housing expert and former chair of Hanover Housing Association. 'In England, 4.2 million pensioners own properties with two bedrooms they don't use.[8] If just 2 per cent of them moved out, this could free up 85,000 homes for families who need houses with gardens. Do that every year for ten years and we could house 4 million people!'

I first met the ebullient Lord Best, who is 73, when I worked in Downing Street and was pondering the UK's housing crisis. Given the very slow rate of housebuilding, and planning restrictions in a densely populated country, it seemed to me that persuading older people to downsize was an obvious way to free up properties for the young. In Britain, around two-thirds of over-65s own their homes outright.[9] Many of those are large family homes with empty bedrooms which are costly to heat, and gardens which are tough on creaky knees.

Surveys suggest that at least a quarter of those people would like to downsize. This would free up some of the enormous unmortgaged housing wealth held by the over-60s – estimated to be around £1.2 trillion in England alone.[10] But attractive alternatives are needed. Councils could zone sites specifically for downsizers, and help with paperwork and moving. And governments could offer tax breaks for moving, or help with renovating, sorting through and moving 50 years' worth of belongings, which can be a big psychological barrier.

Ultimately, we need far more options. While some need to downsize, others find their large family houses are starting to fill up again – with returning adult children. The financial crash and its aftermath have made multi-generational living a financial necessity.

One English couple I know built a 'granny flat' in the basement for themselves to move into, when they could no longer manage the stairs. It is now a 'graddy flat', occupied by their two sons, who've graduated from university. In England, where students have had to pay university tuition fees since 1998, nearly half of those who graduated in 2015 are back living with their parents.[11]

Over 60 million Americans are now living in households which include two or more adult generations.[12] In 2014, for the first time in 130 years, more 18 to 34-year-olds were living with parents than in any other living arrangement.[13]

It's not yet clear whether this phenomenon will fade, as economies pick up and people feel more financially secure, or whether multi-generational living will become an active choice. Retooling homes to incorporate more people is an exciting possibility. In California, the developer Nex Gen has had success with its 'two homes, one price' deals: you get a house, plus a smaller apartment next door. Moving an aged parent or a student child next door keeps them close, but avoids bumping into them in the bathroom.

The New Kinds of Family

Paradoxically, many older people are more isolated than ever before. Not least because divorce and remarriage have changed the shape of the extended family into one which cannot always fit emotionally, let alone physically, beneath a single roof.

One answer is to create a new version of the extended family – just not necessarily your own. In Germany, government-funded *Mehrgenerationenhauser* ('multi-generational houses') incorporate nurseries, homework clubs and elder care centres in open-plan sites. There is a great deal of intermingling, with open doors between great-grandmothers, toddlers and single parents who struggle to balance childcare and work. An imaginative Grandparents' Service

(*Grosselterndienst*) matches older people with single parents to help with babysitting and give emotional support.

In Singapore, the government has just opened the first of ten housing developments which will combine flats for older people with facilities for younger ones: including a kindergarten, playground and childcare centre. The schemes are called 'Kampung', after the old, traditional village compounds, which were lost when Singapore's Housing Development Board built public housing to get people out of slums in the 1950s. The Board has also started to build larger flats which can house three generations of a family, hoping to renew the tradition of relatives and neighbours looking out for each other.

Some of the best schemes are being pioneered by social entrepreneurs who can see how things are changing in Extra Time. In Australia, a brilliant organisation called HomeShare connects older people with a spare room, to students who need somewhere to live, in exchange for ten hours a week of chores.

In Dublin, an older man called John offered student Amy his spare room after he lost his wife. John felt he would like someone else around the house and that he would welcome some help with cooking. He says he has been 'delighted' to feel that he's not alone. Amy was living in a cramped two-room bungalow with six other students and was having to fight to use the stove, with arguments over the electricity meter taking a toll on her university grades. 'John's got a wicked sense of humour,' she told Ireland TV. 'You warm to him straight away, he's just fantastic to live with and his whole family have been so supportive.' Amy and John have lived together for two years through HomeShare. This is a very practical way to combat loneliness, which relies not on charity but good old-fashioned reciprocity.

Stereotypes about the generations not wanting to mix may be completely wrong. Nowhere did I see that more clearly than in the Netherlands.

You're Never Too Old (Or Young) to Be a Good Neighbour

Walking into the Humanitas Deventer retirement home, two hours east of Amsterdam, feels like entering a raucous coffee shop. There's no eerie hush, no wilting pot plants or old folk huddled around a TV. Instead, there's a riot of colour and noise. Five elderly people are chatting in a bar area, under funky coloured lamps. Two toddlers stand entranced by a knee-high robot called Faro, which is travelling slowly along the bright green carpet, singing 'Je Ne Regrette Rien'. A 20-year-old student is controlling the robot from an orange sofa, grinning at the surprised faces of two old ladies nearby.

Six university students live here with 160 elderly people aged between 79 and 100. They get rent-free accommodation in return for spending 30 hours a month with the residents: helping with chores, giving computer lessons or just making conversation. One student lives on each corridor; walking through the garden, I can tell which rooms are theirs by looking at the beer crates stacked on their balconies. The elderly residents come to life hearing about the students' exams and relationships; they especially love dissecting events the morning after, when new girlfriends are sometimes spotted trying to slip away by the fire escape.

'Before I came I would only see the limitations,' says student Sores Duman, a short, wiry guy with a beatific smile and heavy stubble, who has lived here for two years. 'I saw only the things they couldn't do. But now, I see endless possibilities.' Sores is doing a degree in communications and hopes to work in PR. He shows me the tattoo on his left shoulder with the name of his dance group: 'All of the Above'. He recently won a TV game-show prize for break dancing. His main surprise, on arriving at the home, was that the residents 'still have so much life in them'. He loves to party: 'When I throw parties, the elderly come but they get tired and leave at 9 p.m. They're a bit deaf, they can't hear the music late at night from their rooms, so they don't mind. Everyone is so easy-going.' Do his friends think coming here is a bit odd? 'No, they all know how it is.' And his apartment is 'better than a lot of student rooms – I get everything to myself, my own kitchen and bathroom'.

One of the first residents Sores got to know was Marty, 91, who needed help with her iPad. The IT sessions soon developed into long conversations about families. 'She was very interested in where I'm from. When she found out I was Kurdish she looked it all up and we talk about it,' he says. Marty told him about her experiences in the Second World War. He pops round twice a week to have a chat. 'I look at her now and I no longer see a 91-year-old woman but my good friend who has many different parts to her life.'

This is a place where real relationships are built. Not the kind of one-shot activity, where schoolchildren visit to sing a song, but deeper friendships which develop over time. It used to be common to grow up with your grandparents around. But now, societies are having to fill the gap.

'There was one student who gave a party, there were three drunken girls in his room and a bra lying in the hallway,' says Gea Sijpkes, the director of Humanitas. 'The next day at breakfast the residents were all gossiping and forgot about their bad knees.' Staff were less pleased. But when a nurse was attacked by a troubled lady with dementia one night, staff woke up Jurien, a student who had been teaching the woman to use a computer. 'When she saw me,' he says, 'she instantly relaxed.' He spent the rest of the night with her, keeping her calm and watching movies, before cycling off to class.

In leopard-skin ankle boots and a black wrap dress, blonde hair swept back in a bun, Gea Sijpkes could pass for a former Bond girl. She ushers me up a brightly carpeted slope, which I soon realise is a camouflaged wheelchair ramp. A grey-haired lady walking down takes my arm, all smiles, and starts telling me something about her *'vader'*. 'This is Gerrie, she lives two floors down from her father,' explains Gea, embracing Gerrie, who sighs happily and repeats: 'two'. 'Gerrie is 73 and her father is 91. She wasn't happy where she

was living, so we brought her here,' says Gea, with no further explanation. That's what happens at Humanitas: they solve problems.

When Gea became director in 2012 she set out to create 'the
warmest, nicest house where every elderly person wants to live'. It
can't have been easy. The building is an ugly 1960s block with lino-
leum staircases and the budget is the same as at any other state-
funded care home. Most of the residents here are working class; they
are not paying top-up fees.

'I tried to imagine what it would be like to know the doctors can't
repair you,' says Gea. 'When you're elderly you have grief, you have
lost friends and relations. We can't change those facts. But we can
make a warm environment. I want a smile a day, not just a pill. I
wanted people to have experiences of their own, not just wait for
their grandson to visit. I thought, what can I do to liven it up?'

She painted the hallways in crazy colours, put polystyrene flowers
on the walls of the dementia unit to dampen noise and coated whole
doors in photographs of street scenes so that dementia sufferers would
not realise when they were locked in. But she was also determined to
break down the walls between the home and the world outside. She
tried but failed to persuade local schools to use the facilities so she
told her board she wanted university students to live at the home.

'They said students are about sex, drugs, rock'n'roll, they can't
live with vulnerable old people. They even thought students might
sexually abuse the elderly,' she says, pouting. 'Why would they think
that? The students are very nice young people growing up to become
beautiful adults. And the elderly are not vulnerable – they raised
their own children, lived their own lives, now we treat them as voice-
less,' she declares defiantly, her blue eyes sharp.

This belief that the elderly are still individuals, with independent
voices and characters, not just bodies to be tended, is a fundamental
part of the Humanitas vision. The old people here are called 'neighbours', not patients or residents. This emphasises the feeling of home
and of helping one another.

The Board eventually agreed to let one student in, Onno Selbach. He was the only person at the local college who answered Gea's advert. Gea told him there would be just one rule: to be a 'good neighbour'. Onno, a social work student, stacked his bedroom with beer and initially upset staff by sometimes staggering home tipsy in the early hours. But he soon made friends with the residents and became very close to some, including one 93-year-old man, who liked to tell him war stories.

Six years later, and the scheme is oversubscribed. I sit in the dining room watching the newest recruit, Yvonna, 22, who has just beaten 40 other applicants to the one vacant student apartment. In blue shirt and black leather trousers, hair in a ponytail, she is rushing around handing out napkins to about 25 eager elderly people who have propelled themselves here in their motorised scooters for the 'bread meal': the traditional working-class tea at which a student helps out every day.

Did she find it daunting, coming to live with people 60 years her senior? 'Not at all,' she smiles demurely. 'It feels so natural, everyone is 100 per cent themselves. And I wanted to be useful,' she murmurs, before running over to pick up someone's knife from the floor. The old folk twinkle at her every move.

'The students bring the outside world in,' says Gea. 'They have conversations that are much more like everyday life than when they are only a group of elderly people talking. Then it is mainly about illnesses, or that somebody has died. Now they are talking about the break-dancing prize that Sores has won!'

Only one student has so far been asked to leave – I'm told he kept himself to himself too much. The others have brought in new ideas. I meet Harry TerBraak, a dapper gentleman of 91 who used to be a hairdresser and has a beautifully neat apartment. He tells me about making salads with two students, Patrick and Jurien, who created the wild flower garden outside, where the elderly can pick flowers. He explains that he has been advising Patrick on how to grow vegetables and on the importance of hygiene. 'With the students we are among equals,' he says. 'They don't treat us as if we are old.'

The more time I spent at Humanitas, the more I reflect that if you're not treated as 'old' – as somehow apart from everyone else – you probably don't feel so old. I am shown the small gym, where residents and students can cycle on an exercise bike with a virtual reality screen so you can imagine you are in the mountains. Gea tells me about coming to work one morning to find hundreds of green balloons floating all over the home, blown up by students for a laugh. 'Why not?' she says, smiling, and I feel yes, why not? Elderly people have a sense of humour, a sense of fun, like everyone else. 'I know their names,' says Gea, 'I know where they laugh from.'

Humanitas Deventer feels less like an institution than any care home I have ever visited. Attention is paid to the little things: colourful teacups decorated by staff and residents, friendly corners where people can cook and eat together, a beautiful table made from local wood chosen by residents. And it is doing all of this at a time of cutbacks.

'We realised we couldn't afford the welfare state we created after the war, where everyone over 80 could get an inclusive ticket in a place like this,' Gea explains. In 2012, the year she became director, the Dutch government stopped funding continuing care for citizens over the age of 80, unless they were in dire need. 'The cuts,' says Gea, 'made me re-think what business I was in. I decided I was in the happiness business.' They also gave her the opportunity to rewrite the rules. 'If all you do is stay within the regulations,' she says, 'what's the point?' Before she took over, one manager tells me, new arrivals had to fill out a form containing almost 100 questions. Now there are only three: Who are you? Who were you? And who are you going to be?

Who are you *going* to be? How rarely is anyone over the age of 30 asked a question like that, let alone the 80-year-olds who Gea Sijpkes is asking. Her hopes for them, her belief that everyone deserves to be happy until the end of life, are self-fulfilling. It's hardly surprising that this home is now oversubscribed, by middle-class people who have traditionally preferred the more luxurious places near the river. They know that money doesn't matter as much as vision.

Even if we need help in our later years, we shouldn't have to give up on who we are, or on participating in the world.

The 'Young-Old' Commune

Andrea Hargreaves, 71, has made what her children consider to be a deeply impetuous decision: she has sold her house and moved in with two other ladies at the same stage of life. Sallie-Mae is a 65-year-old artist that Andrea met in the local choir, and Lyn, 66, is a retired fashion expert, who recently moved back from Spain. 'Don't tell my children,' Andrea laughs, 'but I didn't even know them that well.'

The two divorcees and one widow, all grandmothers, have sold their two semis and one terraced house to buy a large Edwardian house with a big garden on the Sussex coast in England.

A few days before we speak, the group held a New Year's Eve party which, Andrea tells me, went on until quarter past three in the morning. 'How many people did you have?' I ask. 'Oh, about 40,' she says casually. In September, they organised two weekends where they displayed pictures by local artists, played live music and even hosted a sculpture workshop in the garden. They're planning to do it again this year.

Does she feel old? 'No. I don't have any aches and pains,' she says. Her mother lives five minutes away. 'When you have a mother who is 96, it rather throws your status as an elderly person out of the picture. Why have a label? We've been very lucky. We are the first generation to be able to style ourselves young, and we can believe it – at least until we catch sight of ourselves in a mirror.'

The move to the new house was a grown-up decision, not a whim. The ladies drew up a joint declaration of trust and carefully defined what each of them needs to be happy. For Lyn, a keen vegetable grower, it was the huge garden, which takes three of them to manage. For Sallie-Mae, it was having a studio for her art. Andrea, a retired journalist, wanted all her furniture to be used. Her late husband didn't quite share her sense of style, she says, and she had got some comfort from finding things from junk shops after he died.

Their kind of communal living isn't for everyone. A fourth friend pulled out, after deciding she couldn't face sharing a kitchen. But for the three, the adventure has been rejuvenating.

'Living together seems to make our energy grow,' says Andrea. 'When you live on your own you get home and shut the baked potato in the oven and open a tin of baked beans. You can't do that when you're duty-bound to provide a decent meal for the others three times a week.' She has done things, she says, she would never have attempted on her own – like hosting the weekend festivals and keeping chickens. These are very much on her mind when we speak, because they keep escaping. It sounds like the three women had a hilarious time, rounding them up and wrestling them back into the coop.

'Has the group thought about what could happen if any of them become frail?' I ask.

'We tried to discuss it, but we couldn't get beyond the idea of a carer in the spare room. I'm not sure it would be practical to have one carer for three doddery old ladies and we don't have space for more. But you don't know. You could get your crystal ball out, but frankly, I don't worry about it. I didn't worry about what was going to happen before, so why should I start now?'

Living It Up

The 'Young-Old' do not want a quiet life, they want to live like they mean it. The 'Old-Old' do not wish to be warehoused and bossed around, they want to remain the authors of their own lives.

What everyone needs is a neighbourhood, preferably designed with their input. The clear health benefits from social connections and community mean that it should be in the interest of governments to facilitate co-housing and to bolster membership organisations (Southwark Circle closed in 2014, due to government cuts).

No one yet knows quite how the multi-generational family will affect the way we live. But what is clear is that both young and old will increasingly want to live in cities where there is access to jobs, training courses, the arts and hospitals. In 2007, for the first time in history, half of the world's population was living in urban areas. By 2050 that is expected to reach 70 per cent.[14] A nascent movement for 'age-friendly cities' is developing to drive change. New York has added 1,500 new benches for people to sit on, near community facilities. In Copenhagen, a wonderful scheme called Cycling Without Age transports older people around in free rickshaws. And these changes are coming not a moment too soon. In Lisbon and Milan, women over 75 are the single largest age group.[15] There are literally millions of older people in European cities who rarely or never leave their homes for social, emotional, financial or mobility reasons. It's no good having a 'kneeling' bus if you can't get to the bus stop – or you're scared to walk down the street because it's unsafe.

Living longer does not have to mean being institutionalised and being 'done to'. It should entail being part of a neighbourhood, with the support and attention of other human beings. However well we age, we need other people around us. And while intelligent technology will help look out for us, it is still humans who need to respond, as we will see in the next chapter.

8

Health Revolution

Robots care for you, humans care about you

MOST DAYS, JANE GETS in her car and drives to front doors without knowing what she will find behind them. Yesterday, it was a lady who'd come out of hospital after a long illness and was too wobbly to have a shower on her own. Today, it's a 90-year-old man who is grateful to see her, but embarrassed, as he can't get out of bed without help. Tomorrow, it will be an 80-year-old woman with dementia, clad in a violent pink dressing gown, flapping dangerously open, who will keep asking, 'Where's Mary?'

Jane has taken over Mary's cases, because Mary has left the agency. She will look through the medical folder in the living room of the woman with the violent pink dressing gown. Here, the revolving cast of characters who visit – the district nurse, other care workers, a social worker – are supposed to write updates. Jane will read what medications the woman is taking, but she isn't allowed to dispense them so she will look for clues about this frightened woman. She will ask her about the photos on the mantelpiece, to try to establish a relationship. She will look in the fridge, to see if the woman is eating. And pretty soon, she will have to leave again, to get to her next client.

Jane has some regulars. One, an elderly man she likes very much, was recently in darkness when she arrived, because the light had broken in the bedroom. Jane got a ladder and changed the bulb, knowing she was breaking health and safety rules. But how else was he going to get light? She thinks it's madness that she's not allowed to give medication – his wife used to do it before she died, and she wasn't qualified. It's rules and restrictions everywhere, with too little room for kindness.

Jane is one of the brave, unacknowledged frontline workers holding together a broken system. A system in which carers like her are sent to people's houses for sometimes as little as 15 minutes a day, with minimal training, because the state cannot pay for more. They are poorly paid, sometimes on zero hours contracts with no job security.

Jane says there is not enough time to care, to build a relationship. She is thinking about going back to book-keeping. Every year, 30 per cent of care workers like her leave the system in England, meaning agencies have to spend even more to train and recruit.[1] And the old people are back on the merry-go-round of strange faces.

I first met Jane in 2013 when the Secretary of State for Health asked me to conduct an independent review into the skills and careers of junior nursing and care staff.[2] I travelled round England and Wales, interviewing workers who are largely invisible to the public. Many were compassionate, committed middle-aged women – with a sprinkling of resilient, dedicated men – who said that no one outside their trade union had ever asked for their views before. They spoke of elderly people falling through gaps in a system which is divided between GPs, hospitals and community services, with little information flowing between. They talked about how they were often ignored by senior doctors, nurses and managers, and how they struggled to afford the car insurance and petrol they needed to do their jobs.[3]

Care work is undervalued, underpaid, emotionally draining and physically exhausting. Yet it is, in my view, highly skilled. It requires enormous maturity and resilience; deep wells of kindness too. As

populations age, we are going to need more carers with those qualities, not least because the new Holy Grail of healthcare, in every
high-income country, is keeping people out of hospitals. If someone
lives with heart problems for 20 years, it's prohibitively costly to
whisk them onto a ward every time they have a scare. Instead, we
want to keep them in what is fondly called 'the community'.

Trouble is, we're not very good at it. Too many people find themselves pinging between different medical silos, with long waits,
having to repeat their story every time. And there is an almost total
disconnect, in the UK, US and many other countries, between the
health service and long-term 'social care' – help with things like
washing, dressing, or eating. In the UK, the NHS is free but most
people pay for 'social care'. In the US, Medicare will reimburse for
hospital and physician expenses, but not for long-term care.

A few years ago, I met an 89-year-old gentleman who had made a
note of every carer who had crossed his threshold in the previous
year. He showed me the list: there were 102 names on it. Some had
only come once, then vanished – probably into a better-paying job at
the local supermarket. That is the stark reality of how little we value
our elderly.

Luckily, there is a better way.

The Power of Dutch Kindness

I'm climbing the stairs of an apartment block in Den Haag, the
Netherlands, with Nurse Josie. It's a cold March day and the low-lying
clouds are Vermeer grey. Josie, a sturdy lady in her fifties with a wide,
teddy-bear face, is puffing a bit as we head for the third floor. But what
worries me is that panting behind us are Josie's two Border Terriers.
I cannot imagine any home-care service in England allowing a nurse
to take two small, hairy dogs to a client visit. What about hygiene?

Josie is telling me about the old lady, Berit, who we are going to
visit. Berit has early-stage dementia and can get agitated. Apparently,
she is looking forward to trying out her English on me, as she used

to work in a souvenir shop. I nod, but I'm less concerned about my lack of Dutch than the dogs scampering at our heels. Is this really a good idea?

When we reach the third floor and the door opens, I realise that the dogs are our secret weapon. Berit, 93, stooped and pouting in a yellow fleece and bare feet, initially looks uncertain. Then she sees the dogs and smiles. The terriers have obviously been here before; they rush in and roll ecstatically on the carpet. Once I've been introduced, sipped coffee and exchanged jokes about the Tower of London, Josie hands Berit a plastic bag full of dog treats. Berit rises slowly to her feet, concentrating hard and fishing about in the bag with long, pale fingers. She carefully selects two treats of identical size as the little dogs sit at her feet, tails wagging expectantly. When they take the treats, her face breaks into a huge smile.

This is what happens when you put humanity before bureaucracy. This is Buurtzorg, a Dutch model of care which lets nurses – not some remote, cost-cutting manager – decide what is right for each of their patients. Not everyone likes dogs; Josie's stay obediently in the car on many visits, but she knows that they make Berit happy, calm and more willing to let Josie in. As Berit shows me photos of her trip to London in 1978, I can see out of the corner of my eye that Josie is quietly checking the fridge and dishes to see if Berit has remembered to eat. Her dementia is making her forgetful but also angry. Last week, she started shouting at cars when she was trying to cross the road to the local shop. Her son Bruno is worried; he can only visit at weekends. Josie logs Berit's mood on the Buurtzorg app which Bruno can see, on the iPad which Buurtzorg issues to all its nurses.

Buurtzorg issues iPads, but few commands. Unlike every other care service I've ever encountered, there are no tick sheets or timetables. Nurses work in local teams of no more than 12, and are expected to assess clients, organise their own schedules and even find their own office space: Josie's team operates from two small rooms at the foot of a concrete block containing four chairs, two desks, a filing cabinet and a dog bed. They don't need anything bigger, they tell me, because they want to be out visiting people, not sitting at computers typing reports.

Head office pays the team's rent, sorts out the payroll and handles IT. But it's tiny: only 50 people at HQ support 10,000 Buurtzorg nurses and care assistants. As a result, its overheads are about 8 per cent, compared with 25 per cent for comparable organisations. The money saved is used to employ more nurses, because Buurtzorg is non-profit.

It's hard to explain how revolutionary this is. In so many countries, systems have become dehumanised, hedged about with rules and regulations. Compassion has been downgraded in favour of risk assessments. And no one has time to care.

Buurtzorg was founded in 2007 by a male nurse, Jos de Blok, who had become disillusioned with the Dutch health service. 'Healthcare and community care were defined as production,' he says. 'We defined ten different products: nursing, nursing care extra, guidance extra – for commissioners that's the way they buy care – so many hours of this and so many hours of that.' The resulting relationship between patients and nurses, he has said, 'was really disturbing'.

A well-spoken man in his sixties with greying temples, de Blok started his first team with just three colleagues, aiming to restore meaningful relationships between staff and patients. His philosophy is to 'keep things simple', so 'you don't need so many people to control all these things'. And to remove hierarchies. 'We haven't had one management meeting since we started,' he says. 'My old job was only about meetings. Now we have time to solve the problems.' And it's working. Today, Buurtzorg serves 70,000 patients across the Netherlands. Nurses have come out of retirement to join it, so enthusiastic are they about the philosophy.

Back in Berit's flat, the Tower of London photographs have been put aside and I'm now drowning under an album of her 1980 trip to Berlin. Josie has decided not to apply the cream for Berit's psoriasis until tomorrow, because to undress her now would disrupt a conversation which she is enjoying. Berit is a wonderfully forceful character – telling me stories of the past in a halting mixture of Dutch and English – but she sometimes loses her thread, her shoulders stoop and her bare feet look painfully warped on the thick carpet.

It's time for the next appointment. 'You're leaving the dogs here?' I ask Josie as we say our goodbyes. 'Yes,' she says confidently, 'I'll collect them later. You can see the light in her eyes, can't you?' she whispers proudly, catching my scepticism. And I can. Giving Berit the companionship and responsibility of these little dogs is undoubtedly part of what keeps her going.

As I drive around with Josie the rest of the morning, I am struck by three things. First, the continuity of care. In every home we visit there is a booklet with pictures of the only three team members a client will ever see, who are responsible for their care. Second, the emphasis on self-reliance and family networks. Josie and her colleagues are proactive about seeking out friends and family, keeping them informed and getting them involved.

Third, no team member sees any task as beneath them. In the UK, we parcel activities into 'professional' tasks, like giving medication, done by registered nurses, and 'basic' tasks, like helping someone shower, done by care staff. But Josie loves doing it all. She tells me she joined Buurtzorg to connect with patients again. 'I'm going back to my roots, working with people,' she says, with a joyful look. 'We take care of everything – we'll make a sandwich for a client if that's what they need.'

In the UK, I long ago came to the view that our obsessive allocation of tasks to the cheapest member of staff is a false economy. A monstrous bureaucracy is required to oversee it and no one has time to build an actual relationship. This often means that patients deteriorate faster and require more and more help. For the good of patients, we need to start focusing on outcomes, not costs. And we might even, paradoxically, save money.

Buurtzorg seems to prove my theory about efficiency. Despite often paying qualified nurses to do all tasks, which means that the service costs more per hour than comparable agencies, Buurtzorg ends up costing almost 40 per cent less overall, according to the consultancy EY.[4] This is because staff need to put in fewer hours with each patient. And that, in turn, is a result of trust. Josie and her colleagues encourage patients to manage their own conditions and they're good at getting relatives involved to help with that. Patients don't panic and call head office endlessly, because they know Josie is coming back. Buurtzorg, in that sense, is creating neighbourhoods – which, as we have already seen, can improve health.

Josie gives the impression that she has all the time in the world on her visits, but during my morning with her I realise that she is flexing skilfully. We spend only ten minutes with one elderly lady who needs compression socks putting on, but it feels longer, as Josie and the lady are chatting all the while. 'The clients have the feeling that I'll take five or ten minutes extra when they need it,' she says. 'They have the knowledge that we'll be there when they need it.'

Client satisfaction rates for Buurtzorg are higher than for any comparable healthcare organisation in Holland. In fact, Buurtzorg may be making even greater savings for the state, by reducing demand for other services. 'Buurtzorg are my family,' says Anita, a middle-aged lady we meet who is recovering from lung cancer. 'I can tell Josie things I don't want even my sister to know. The hospital doctor asked, did I want to see a counsellor? But I don't know them. Why would I talk to them? I talk to Josie.'

Treating people as human, building proper relationships and paying those who have a vocation, for what I would call the 'craftsmanship' of nursing, may sound like common sense. But in today's world, it's radical.

The problem is most acute in Japan, where the dwindling population has left the government predicting 380,000 care staff vacancies by 2025.[5] To replace and augment human carers, the Japanese government is now investing heavily in technological solutions.

The Robots Are Coming

In Aichi province, central Japan, a loudspeaker blares down the street. It's asking if anyone has seen an 85-year-old lady wearing a bright pink shirt. 'If you see her, please report to the police station,' barks the tinny voice.

Originally put in place to warn of typhoons and earthquakes, Japan's public warning system is now frequently commandeered to search for elderly people with dementia. Mrs Ahote, the lady with the pink shirt, is one of almost 16,000 who go missing each year in Japan. Last year, about 500 of those met with fatal accidents.[6]

At the Shintomi nursing home in Tokyo, Director Yukari Sekiguchi foresees a world in which everyone will have to be monitored electronically, because there are no longer enough children to keep an eye on parents.

'Around here, there are many apartments with elderly citizens living alone,' she says quietly, her eyes full of concern. 'Some will come and visit us for rehabilitation, or to take a bath. But when they go home, we don't know how they survive.' Ms Sekiguchi, a petite, dark-haired lady with beautifully embroidered flowers on her blue shirt, says that her staff recently rescued a 70-year-old woman living alone, who had swallowed two days' worth of pills by mistake. This is, apparently, quite a common occurrence. 'Do they have no relatives to look out for them?' I ask. Ms Sekiguchi shrugs. 'The families live far away,' she says grimly.

Inside Shintomi, where most residents are in their late eighties, Ms Sekiguchi's staff are trying out a range of technologies to keep watch on them when staff can't. During the night, there is only one staff member on each floor of this eight-storey building so each bed has an electronic sensor under the mattress which can pick up a change in someone's breathing pattern. Other sensors detect movement across the floor, alerting night staff if someone gets out of bed.

Similar systems are being developed for use at home. One called Owl Light uses infra-red light, which is felt to be less intrusive than having a fully fledged CCTV camera in every room. But it's clear that ageing is blurring the boundaries of privacy. Anxious relatives hope to monitor, from a distance.

The robots are coming too, driven by a shortage of humans. 'Even now, we prefer robots to Filipinas,' one doctor told me, shaking his head with frustration.

Japan leads the world in these amazing technologies and the Japanese seem very much at ease living alongside them. A five-foot humanoid robot called Pepper, who looks a bit like a white plastic version of C-3PO from *Star Wars*, recently greeted me in the foyer of a Tokyo bank. He was rather endearing, with deep, dark eyes and a high-pitched, giggly voice. In the bank, he was mainly a gimmick which kept us entertained by dancing while we waited in the queue. But in some care centres, Pepper robots are now leading groups of old people in exercise classes.

Watching elderly people being led in a routine by Pepper was a surreal experience. Some of the old ladies had wheeled themselves forward to be closer to him and were avidly copying his arm move-ments. One touched his head and laughed flirtatiously when he addressed her. Others – including the three elderly men in the audi-ence – seemed more interested in eating their lunch.

Experts say that Pepper brings some depressed people out of their shells, helping them to re-engage with the world. A Japanese physio-therapist told me he finds older people are more willing to copy Pepper than human physios in the exercise routines. Ms Sekiguchi, of Shintomi, thinks this may have something to do with his giggly, high-pitched speech patterns. 'Pepper's rhythm seems to fit the elderly, especially those with dementia,' she says.

Another companion robot is RoBoHoN, a 20-centimetre high, plastic black and white figure with a cute, monkey-like face, which can sit on an elderly person's bedside table and make cheery comments to get them out of bed in the morning, telling them that their health has improved or saying, 'It's been a while since you went out, shall we go for a walk?'

RoBoHoN is basically a sophisticated phone which can walk on two legs and uses voice and face recognition. He (everyone refers to RoBoHoN as 'he', it's hard not to) can work out where you are in the room and move towards you.

'Thanks for looking after me, Robby,' says a smiling, grey-haired lady in the marketing video I'm shown at Nagoya University, where scientists are pioneering applications of these technologies. Professor Takayuki Morikawa, at the university, says people often feel more comfortable with RoBoHoN than with more conventional electronic screens.

Robby cannot yet hold a fully fledged conversation, but his creators are working to develop his AI to the point where he will be able to judge your mood – and hence gauge what kind of comments to make – by sensing your stress levels through sensors in your armchair, which will monitor your brain waves.

I can't help wondering if some of us might find our stress levels permanently raised if we had furniture recording our every move and a plastic robot masquerading as a friend. But there's no doubt that these technologies will be a lifeline for those who want to remain independent. Although who knows what will happen in the future if an old person decides to sneak a cigarette, or to download something unsuitable. I've always thought that towards the very end of life, people should grab what pleasures they can. I presume the robots will be programmed to boss them out of such things and to make relentlessly cheerful remarks to turn them onto a better path.

My father used to say that complaining was one of the last pleasures available to the very old. Unlike the stoic Japanese, who look politely surprised when I ask if people will feel comfortable with these gadgets, we Europeans – especially Celts like me – may need robots which can moan. Perhaps Douglas Adams was onto something when he invented Marvin the Paranoid Android in *The Hitchhiker's Guide to the Galaxy* ('Brain the size of a planet and they ask me to pick up a piece of paper ... is that job satisfaction?').

Manufacturers frequently talk about robots sensing our emotions. Softbank Robotics claims that Pepper is 'the first humanoid robot capable of recognising the principal human emotions, and adapting his behaviour to the mood of his interlocutor'. But that doesn't make robots emotional beings. We can't attribute humanity to electronic devices coated in plastic.

Or can we? In her book *Alone Together: Why We Expect More from Technology and Less from Each Other*, the psychologist Sherry Turkle argues that the more we project human qualities onto robots, the more our expectations of other human beings dwindle. 'Sociable robots meet our gaze, speak to us, and learn to recognize us,' Turkle writes. 'They ask us to take care of them; in response, we imagine that they might care for us in return.' One consequence, Turkle fears, is that we stop talking to each other. In particular, we stop listening to what our elderly have to say. Real conversation requires listening to the nuances of what someone is really saying, not just responding with a script to what they literally said.

A mechanical arm doesn't need a face – it's not pretending to understand you, it's just doing a physical job which saves your carer from a back injury. I saw some marvellous ones in Japan, including a bed which turns into a wheelchair while the patient is still in it, which saves endless amounts of backache, and a thick-trunked rehabilitation robot for stroke patients called 'Tree', which you hold on to for support while it helps you learn to walk again. These are miraculous devices and I can only pray that the costs fall enough for them to spread far and wide. Those straying into emotional territory may be trickier for us to accept, but who can deny that they may provide a level of comfort which humans cannot, for those with dementia?

Robot animals are a halfway house. Paro, a furry seal which bats its long eyelashes at you when you stroke it, is frankly irresistible. It's already being used in care homes in Denmark and the US.

I watch, fascinated, as three elderly Japanese ladies stroke their Paros. 'She listens to me,' whispers the first, with a wizened face, who is so tiny she can barely reach the table. 'She responds to me,' she says slowly. The second is sunk in reflection, apparently unaware we are there. The third, a lady with gold-rimmed glasses, is an 82-year-old former golfer. She explains that she prefers Paro to Aibo, the dog robot, because she is a cat person, not a dog person (and Aibo, although it wags its tail appealingly, is not cuddly: it's made of hard grey plastic).

'We had cats until the end of the war,' the ex-golfer recalls wistfully. 'My mother was known as the Cat Lady. Then the famine came, and we couldn't keep them.' Snapping back into the present, she gets impish. 'When I tap her on the face she cries,' she says, showing me how Paro mewls plaintively when she taps it hard. She is clearly aware that Paro is not real. For the other two ladies, reality seems more blurred.

Paro was invented by Takanori Shibata, chief senior research scientist at Tsukuba's National Institute of Advanced Industrial Science and Technology. Shibata chose a seal because people were less familiar with seals than with domestic pets like dogs or cats, so were more likely to bond with a fake version. He went to Canada to watch real seals in action and used recordings of Canadian harp seals to generate Paro's cries. The seal has been shown to reduce anxiety and depression, and even pain during chemotherapy. It is so effective in calming down some dementia patients and stopping them from wandering off that it has even replaced psychotropic drugs in some cases.

Without doubt, these creatures provide a level of comfort which busy humans cannot. And if Japan continues to age at the current rate, there won't be enough humans to listen. Some manufacturers are even making companion robots for children – like Cocotte, a ball with a face which moves spookily as it rolls – on the assumption that parents may be hard at work paying the taxes to support their old age.

The Invisible Army of Family

Whether human or robot, the numbers of professional carers are dwarfed by the sons, daughters, wives, husbands and others who look after an ageing relative. There are 7.6 million of them in the UK, 670,000 of them looking after people with dementia, according to the Carers Trust.[7]

These people are largely invisible. They slog away heroically, leaving last-minute calls for siblings, taking emergency leave from work. Some have to give up their careers altogether. One of those is Shaheen Larrieux. Her story is an extreme example of what many of us face, if a parent gets dementia.

Shaheen was a high-flying executive at a US software company, who returned to England in 2001 for a few months to help her parents solve some problems in the family accountancy business. She ended up staying for the next 18 years.

'A counsellor said to me, "You are your mum's full-time carer,"' she says. 'I was like, what? I hated the word "carer". But I realised then how much I'd given up. As I look back now, I think, where did all those years go?'

A chemical engineering graduate with an MBA, Shaheen had been planning to take a few months off, then start her own business. But she became worried about her mother Hosna, then 54, who was behaving erratically due to a rare and undiagnosed form of dementia (Frontotemporal Dementia (bvFTD)). A tough Bangladeshi woman, her mother had always dealt with VAT for clients. But that changed: 'If she was writing a cheque she would ask me to write it and she would sign. She didn't want to go to the bank any more. The telephone was a disaster, even though she spoke perfect English.'

Her father started to be driven mad by the way her mother would repeat the same questions, banging her cup on the table. As Shaheen took on more and more, she describes poignantly the experience that so many of us face when a parent gets dementia: 'You slowly turn into the parent, and the parent turns into the child.'

This role reversal needs to be more widely understood, I feel. I myself was totally unprepared for it when my mother developed vascular dementia. At first, neither of us understood what was happening. Instead of asking probing medical questions, as I should have done, I resented her inability to remember key moments from my childhood, when she was still able to endlessly recall events from her own. I was upset by hurtful things she would say, which she was later genuinely unable to remember. The beloved only child, I was frankly pretty graceless about stepping up to the plate. My mother remained fiercely independent to the end, not wanting to be a burden, both us still struggling to fathom where the new boundaries were.

For Shaheen, the days turned into months, then years. 'I got sucked into the process,' she says. Whenever she thought about restarting her career, 'something would happen. Someone was financially abusing my mother and money was going missing. I told Dad not to give her a debit card, but they were all frightened of her.' Hosna was becoming aggressive and Shaheen was losing her confidence. To many of her friends in the corporate world, she had become invisible: 'I'd think, here I am with an MBA but what do I have to offer?'

To make matters worse, relatives would not accept her mother was ill. In her culture, Shaheen says, it is expected that an unmarried daughter will look after her parents, so what was all the fuss about?

The diagnosis in 2013 was an immense relief. 'I had kept thinking: why can't I get along with my mother? You walk on eggshells in order not to set them off. I sought help to try and change myself, thinking that I was the problem, but in the end I realised I was dealing with someone who has a brain disease.'

To me, the most heartbreaking aspect of Shaheen's story is how alone she felt. The police would come round, complaining Hosna had been rude to people in the street. Social services wouldn't help. And Shaheen had to work hard to get medical support. 'The hardest thing I've ever done is dealing with different parts of the NHS trying to co-ordinate care,' she tells me. At one point she downloaded and read a framework for continuing care which ran to 170 pages – 'I don't know how most people can follow it.' That is, I'm afraid, a very common experience. Many carers are elderly themselves, exhausted by the struggle and without Shaheen's business acumen.

Shaheen does not complain. Her father died in 2018 and her mother, now 71, is being well looked after by carers. Shaheen gives talks to companies and is an Alzheimer's Research UK Champion. 'What I've learned is there are different routes to happiness. I've met so many interesting people through the Alzheimer's Society. I spent so many years worrying what people thought – but I don't really care now. I have bonded with my mother through such a terrible disease and I will be left with nice thoughts when she passes. And my dad left this earth knowing that my mom was being looked after. I have found some peace. I don't think I could feel at peace if I was still flying around the world, worrying that something might have happened at home.'

I admire Shaheen enormously, but no one should have to suffer such a struggle. We need more Nurse Josies, people who can support families without necessarily supplanting them. We need holidays and respite for the unpaid carers who are cracking under the strain, and support for younger carers who want to restart their careers. And we need properly funded systems for looking after people.

How to Fund Social Care

We don't know which of us will get Alzheimer's, or crippling arthritis, and who will still be tea-dancing at 90. I hope I've convinced you by now that most of us can substantially improve our odds of tea dancing. But we can never rule out bad luck: when it comes to dementia, we are still playing a version of Russian roulette.

As we go into Extra Time, every country needs an equitable way to finance good care. While many OECD countries have universal social insurance systems for acute healthcare, few have such schemes for looking after the 'Old-Old'.[8] The US, which spends so much on healthcare, spends less on long-term care and it's fragmented, making it harder to establish the kind of comprehensive insurance which is, frankly, the only way to cover the uncertain risk of dementia.

Brits are especially wary of insurance systems – we fear the crazy fees and commercialisation of the US. But the Dutch have a wonderful phrase for their (four) insurance systems: 'Solidarity through insurance which is compulsory for all, and available to all.' That sounds more equitable than the current UK system. If you are unlucky enough to get cancer, you'll be treated for free on the NHS. But if you develop dementia, or Parkinson's, or you are just frail, you must pay for your own care until you're pretty much broke. You must rely on means-tested local care services, of highly variable quality.

When I worked for the UK government, the funding of social care was an issue creeping up in our wing mirrors. The charity Age UK was telling us that 1.4 million older people were not getting help to carry out essential tasks such as washing and dressing. There were fears that a care-home chain might go bust. During the 2015 Spending Review, Sir Jeremy Heywood, the Cabinet Secretary, held an urgent meeting in his office to try to thrash out the size of the funding 'gap'. Representatives from the three relevant departments who attended could not agree. At about the 90th minute, one of the officials at the table broke into a forceful and eloquent tirade that care homes were on the brink of collapse, staff demoralised and the sector was in crisis. It was rare for an official to be so blunt, let alone attack the Treasury in the terms in which he did.

We all knew, or thought we knew, that voters didn't want higher taxes. Few voters knew much about social care, but it was starting to affect hospitals. One in ten hospital beds contained an elderly person who was medically fit to be discharged but had nowhere to go: failing social care was pulling the NHS down with it. But while the public were seeing longer queues at the front door of A&E, they were barely aware of the reason: chaos at the exit. That is now changing and the time is ripe for a social insurance scheme of the kind pioneered in Germany and Japan.

Answers from Germany and Japan

'The government realised things had to change,' says Professor Ichisaburo Tochimoto of Sophia University, Japan. He lifts down one of the dusty boxes above the bookshelves in his office and shows me the estimates he helped to make for every province in the 1990s. Penned in neat lines are the numbers of people over 65 in Hokkaido province, what proportion were living alone or with families and an estimate of their future care needs.

'We could see that the special needs figures were going up fastest,' says Tochimoto. 'This was the shadow of dementia.' That shadow overhung everything and it was growing longer. Japan was facing a perfect storm: increasing numbers of bedridden people, more elderly people living alone and care workers themselves getting older. It was also clear that the long-term hospitalisation of elderly people with dementia was catastrophically expensive. People needed to be encouraged to stay at home if at all possible.

Professor Tochimoto and his colleagues learned from Germany, which was also facing a crisis. Germany's mandatory long-term care insurance fund was introduced in 1994, when its care system looked about as frayed as England's does now. The fund was painstakingly crafted to ensure that everyone got something, no one got something for nothing, and everyone put something in. Workers pay a compulsory levy. Employers contribute half of that, on behalf of their staff, and the retired pay in full. The government got cross-party agreement by abolishing means-testing. The deal with voters was clear: you pay more in, but you get more out. The burden is shared and the risk is pooled.

Japan introduced a similar system in 2000, with a national tax paid by workers over 40.

The Japanese have a strong culture of looking after family, not expecting the state to step in, so they wanted a system which would encourage people to save, make the elderly the policyholders and have them bear the cost of premiums, where possible.

The system is pretty comprehensive. It covers home visits, nursing home stays, help with grocery shopping and the leasing of the unglamorous but useful equipment – handrails, wheelchairs, beds – with people paying an additional 10 per cent to use the services. As demand has risen, so have the co-payments. The richest users must now contribute 20 per cent.

Talking to younger Japanese, I found that many seem to have more faith in the long-term care insurance than in their state pensions. One expert told me that his own son no longer pays into his pension. Governments have tinkered too much, he said. They think the pension will have vanished by the time they grow old, but the care scheme seems more stable – and fair. The main challenges are relentlessly rising costs and the reluctance of many to look after their relatives. No one predicted that so many old people would end up alone.

Germany has tried to head off this problem by allowing budgets to be used to pay relatives. This is popular: it recognises the work of family carers and helps bind the generations together. Germany makes childless couples pay more to the fund than those with children, which might feel almost too logical to some, but which voters seem relatively sanguine about.

Whether you're in Germany, Japan or the Netherlands, these schemes are founded on payroll taxes. Translated to the UK, this would mean a rise in national insurance for everyone over 40, including the over-65s, who are currently exempt. Cash-poor but home-owning pensioners could make the payments by releasing equity from their homes to be recouped after death.

While this wouldn't be popular, it would seem to me to be a fair opening gambit. What's needed is grown-up cross-party discussion, plus better health services.

Revolutionising Healthcare

Health systems are still organised to treat yesterday's problems. Our postwar systems still largely geared to fixing one-time illnesses, rather than to predicting, preventing and treating chronic long-term conditions. One aspect of this is that we still seem to be hiring professionals to treat the illnesses of the young, rather than the old. In the US, the number of geriatricians has actually been dropping as the population ages, with many medical students preferring the glamour and better pay of oncology or paediatrics.[9] In the UK, the number of medical schools teaching geriatrics has fallen.[10] Yet these are the doctors we are going to need most – along with district nurses who keep people out of hospital – whose numbers have been steadily falling in both the UK and France.

Arguably, we should be aiming to have as many geriatricians as paediatricians. Elder care has traditionally lacked glamour. After all, who wants to manage decline? But the best geriatricians achieve wonders by administering hope, not pessimism, and seeing the patient as a whole person, not a problematic knee or hip. Those are the people we need to help us shift healthcare towards staying healthy, not just treating illness.

Technology will be transformational. AI can already diagnose some illnesses better than doctors, and can even identify rare genetic disorders simply by analysing the shape of someone's face. A collaboration between the company Deepmind and Moorfields Eye Hospital in London in 2018 used AI to identify over 50 eye diseases with 94 per cent accuracy. Doctors say this will reduce the risk of sight loss, by significantly reducing the time taken for patients to be diagnosed and treated. That's particularly relevant to Extra Time, because longer lives will increase the number of eye problems.

Machine learning has life-saving potential, as the volume and complexity of medical scans outpaces the availability of humans to interpret them. The Moorfields trial showed that AI can interpret 3D structures, not just 2D images.

Simpler technologies can also liberate busy professionals to spend more time with patients. Nurses who currently spend hours on the phone, ringing up care homes to find places for patients who are well enough to be discharged, could have software which immediately shows where places are free. Voice recognition can cut down the time needed to access patient data. A system of barcode tracking called Scan4Safety is being used in some English hospitals to track all treatments and manage medical supplies, and is forecast to save up to £800 million for the NHS. 'Wearable tech', embedded in clothes or wristbands, can monitor vital signs and beam the information to the clinic. Moreover, genetic testing is likely to become much more widespread: with genomics holding out the promise of using our DNA to find the most effective medicines, tailored to our individual make-up.

All of these changes raise challenges: not least in terms of cybersecurity and data protection. Staff will need to become more literate in digital technologies: a 2018 review by the US academic Eric Topol found that nine in ten jobs in the NHS will require some element of digital skills within 20 years. But as long as we don't delegate everything to robots, technology offers the chance to take more responsibility for our own health, streamline bureaucratic systems and relieve some of the burden on professionals. We are still going to need compassionate carers and we need to value them too.

The Second-Best Time Is Now

One mark of a civilised society, in my opinion, is how it looks after its 'Old-Old'. Yet our health and care systems have become so complex, so rigged with rules and regulations, they sometimes lose sight of the fact that they are dealing with human beings. The Dutch Buurtzorg model demonstrates that kindness, trust and effective care do not have to be bankrupting or inhuman.

Dementia is the most common reason for needing long-term care. People with dementia make up around four-fifths of all those in care homes worldwide[11] and they need intense help. While robots will relieve some of the burden, this can't be done on the cheap. The type of compulsory, comprehensive insurance funds in Germany and Japan are the fairest way to share the burden and reduce risk.

Each of us will need to take more responsibility for our own health, to stay as strong and independent as possible. Many of us, like Shaheen, will care for our parents. We must be prepared to pay a bit more tax to fund a better old age.

There is an old Dutch saying, quoted by one of my husband's Dutch relatives: '*De beste tijd om een boom te planten was 20 jaar geleden. De tweede beste tijd is nu.*' In other words, 'The best time to plant a tree was 20 years ago. The second-best time is now.' It is the responsibility of my generation – Generation X – to lay the foundations for a new era of decent, equitable health and care systems.

9

Finding *Ikigai*

Purpose Is Vital

EXTRA TIME SHOULD BE a gift. Yet time can hang heavy on us, if we don't know what to do with it. When half of all 75-year-olds say the TV is their main form of company,[1] something has gone disastrously wrong: we are out of kilter with ourselves.

Through our human ingenuity, scientific breakthroughs and medical care, we have created an entirely new stage of life: the stage of 'Young-Old'. Now we need to figure out what to do with it.

The longer I have spent researching this book, the more convinced I have become that we humans need purpose, to live fulfilling lives. When someone resigns or retires, or children grow up and leave home, it can rob them of a profound sense of meaning they have relied on, often without thinking. Many retired people I have interviewed have described the sense of falling off a cliff, floundering to find themselves, even if they initially welcomed more leisure. People who have climbed every ladder life presented, bravely meeting challenges along the way, suddenly find themselves with no more rungs to climb and no compass. What is supposed to be a pleasant time of life can be quietly traumatic. That is why I feel so strongly that older people should not be made to give up work and that we must challenge the narrative of 'golden' early retirement. And especially that we need to seek new ways to re-skill and re-engage.

The MacArthur Study of Successful Aging found that people who felt useful in their seventies were significantly less likely to develop health problems or die than those who didn't.[2] A study by Harvard's School of Public Health[3] suggests that physical agility – grip strength and walking speed – is highly correlated with having a strong sense of purpose. Rush University Medical Center has even suggested that those who score highly on a ten-point test for purposefulness are 2.4 times more likely to remain free of Alzheimer's disease, over a seven-year period.[4] None of this is categorical, but it is indicative.

One explanation is that a sense of purpose reduces stress. Another is that purposeful people tend to be more active and look after their health. Either way, it seems intuitively true that having a sense of direction and meaning in our lives can help protect against loneliness, against illness, even against pain.

'Oh well,' says my next-door neighbour Ursula, who is 86 and suffering from back pain, 'I've got to keep going. We're putting on a marvellous concert tomorrow and the students need me.' Ursula is a widow. She has no children but many friends. She cycles everywhere and is passionate about music, and endlessly curious about the world. I bump into her on the street and she says, 'We must get together. But I'm so busy!'

Few people I have interviewed for this book seemed happier than the very elderly Japanese ladies I met in the Edogawa Silver Centre (see page 74). Yes, they enjoy the companionship and gossip from what is a form of coffee morning, but they also feel useful: doing real work for local businesses. There is a genuine reason to show up every day, and to keep going.

Maybe we miss a trick when we invent tea parties to bring older people together. People can be desperately lonely, yet still be reluctant to be shoe-horned into events with others with whom they have nothing in common, except age. Rather than aimless coffee mornings, perhaps we need tea parties with a purpose.

At one day care centre I visited on the south coast of England, struggling to make conversation with an old lady, I said brightly, 'I bet you're looking forward to the bingo.' 'Bloody bingo!' she responded. 'I hate bingo! But that's all they offer.' How patronising of me to have assumed that just because her hair was white, she would enjoy the same game as everyone else. And how blinkered of the organisers.

The Japanese Silver Centres are guided by the concept of *ikigai*, or 'reason for being': literally 'life (*iki*) – purpose (*gai*)', which is so important to the Okinawans. One way of looking at Extra Time could be to say that we should focus on discovering our *ikigai* – on what will keep getting us up in the morning.

Many of us struggle to translate *ikigai* properly, because it seems so at odds with Western hedonism. For many Japanese, it represents a fusion of the spiritual and practical. It connects work, family, duty and passions – it doesn't separate them. *Ikigai* is often said to come at the intersection of four things:

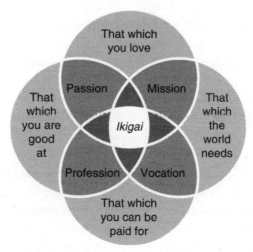

Drawing a Venn diagram like the one above, can make it look like any other career challenge. But at the intersection, you find inner peace. That means dropping the 'shoulds' and the 'oughts'. For those of us raised in a Western tradition, this is not an easy concept. 'I feel so guilty on Monday mornings,' a 76-year-old grandfather recently told me, when we were both picking up our small charges from primary school. 'Everyone else is going to work.' This man plays many useful roles, including being a hands-on grandfather, but he still feels guilty about dropping the commute.

Some retired people are struggling, perhaps too hard, to invent a grand new narrative for their lives. Others derive deep contentment from the small things: singing in a choir, or doing the shopping for a neighbour. My Japanese friend Dora, who is one of the calmest people I know, advises that it is better to ask 'What gives meaning to my life?' than to strain for 'What is my higher purpose?' It's about gratitude, she says, not ambition.

How do we find that purpose? For many people as they grow older, it comes from helping others.

The Park Bench Grandmothers in Zimbabwe

Early in his career as a psychiatrist in his native Zimbabwe, Dixon Chibanda lost a patient. She had been due to come to Harare to see him at the hospital, but didn't show up. A few days later, he got a message: she had hung herself from a mango tree.

Dr Chibanda was terribly distressed. 'Why didn't she come to see me?' he asked her mother. The answer horrified him: she couldn't afford the bus fare.

At that moment, Dr Chibanda realised he needed to radically rethink his job. As one of only five psychiatrists in a nation of 10 million people, he could never hope to meet the overwhelming needs of his country unless he took his work outside the hospital and recruited many more helpers. But who else could he recruit to counsel people in the villages?

The answer: grandmothers.

Grandmothers had the three qualities Dr Chibanda most needed: strong listening skills, empathy and an ability to reflect. So he started off with 14 grandmothers who were already working as community volunteers in the suburb of Mbare, where his own grandmother lived. He trained them in talking therapies and created what became known as the 'Friendship Bench': a park bench where they could sit, out in the open, waiting to give friendly, compassionate advice.

Listening is paramount. When someone sits down on the bench, the first thing the grandmother will say is 'I'm here for you, would you like to share your story with me?' If she thinks someone is suicidal, she alerts the hospital. Otherwise, she will meet the person six times for one-to-one therapy sessions.

Chibanda's team tried putting other kinds of people on the bench: men and younger women. But the grandmothers were better. In fact, they turned out to be even more effective at treating depression than qualified doctors. Six months after leaving the Friendship Bench, people treated there had a lower incidence of anxiety and depression than those who had experienced standard care.[5]

After the first clinical trials, Chibanda's team ran out of funding. They feared the grandmothers would give up. But they kept going, because they believed in the work and they were fulfilled by it. When the team analysed the grandmothers' own mental health, they found it was far higher than they would have expected – probably, they concluded, as a consequence of doing this work, which brought them into contact with new people and gave them an important role in the community.

There are now Friendship Benches in 70 communities in Zimbabwe.[6] On each one sits a grandmother: ready to listen, understand and advise, with Chibanda's training but also with the deep wisdom of her years.

Grandmothers are still deeply respected in Africa. In the West, if we want our ageing societies to keep progressing, we need to harness that same kind of wisdom. After all, we've seen in this book that our brains can stay sharp and make new connections throughout life – and that many pensioners are healthier and more energetic than any generation before. As Marc Freedman, the social entrepreneur and founder of Encore.org, has said, 'Our ageing population is our only increasing natural resource'. So let's use it.

Doing Good Makes You Feel Good

In Baltimore, Maryland, a group of determined people in the 1990s were concerned about the number of children failing and dropping out of school. They knew that what happens before third grade is crucial, but that teachers were stretched to the limit. Like Dixon Chibanda in Zimbabwe, they looked around to see if there was any other resource available and alighted on local older people. They designed a volunteer scheme, in which older adults would intensively tutor children, in literacy, maths and other school priorities, and mentor them too. It was a big commitment. The 15 to 20 volunteers in each school had to spend at least 15 hours a week there for the whole school year.[7]

Being far-sighted, the group – which included a dynamic young geriatrician called Linda P. Fried and was associated with the Johns Hopkins University School of Medicine – designed the roles to be challenging for the adults too. Fried was convinced that there were connections between physical and mental health and purpose. She had been advising some of her older patients to 'find something meaningful to do' – but was dismayed when they reported that they couldn't find anywhere to use their skills. The Baltimore experimenters hoped that their programme might promote cognitive health in ways which reflect some of the early thinking about the brain covered in Chapter 5.

The project was a success.[8] There was a stunning 30 to 50 per cent decline in the number of children referred to the principal's office for behavioural problems. Teachers reported that the presence of so many older people changed the climate in the classroom and the scope of possibilities for all students.

Involvement in the programme improved the physical and mental health of the volunteers compared with their peers, partly because they were more physically active.[9] Brain scans of some volunteers suggested that the experience also improved their problem-solving abilities.

The experiment became a permanent scheme called Experience Corps, which now runs in 22 American cities.[10] A study[11] examining the performance of almost 900 second and third graders in three cities found that those children who had been supported by Experience Corps achieved 60 per cent more progress in reading comprehension than comparable students: a similar effect to halving the class size.

What's surprising is how few schemes like this exist around the world. As populations age, the pressures on public services are rising. There are fewer younger people available to be teachers, nurses and playground supervisors yet at the same time we are awash with older people with time and experience. Why not put the two together? There could be better outcomes for the young and reduced demands on health services for the old.

Volunteers come in many shapes and sizes, and some have surprised themselves by the impact they have.

The HelpForce in England

Bob Groves,[12] 77, has an infectious smile when he greets me in the large English hospital where he works. In repose, his face looks a little pinched, introspective under his slicked-back, dark hair. I spot him as I enter the building, sitting in the large atrium, unaware I am there. But when he sees me and grins, his whole face lights up. I can see why he is so popular with the staff here, and the patients to whom he brings cups of tea.

Bob started volunteering at this, his local hospital, a year ago. He can't explain quite what drew him to it except that he read an article which listed doctors and nurses as the most trusted professionals in the country and found himself wanting to help. He's never thought of himself as gregarious. In fact, 'I've always seen myself as a loner,' he says. 'I had my own business, even at university.' But here, 'It's the opposite,' he says wonderingly. 'Coming to the hospital has been absolutely wonderful. I am so admiring of the doctors and nurses, it reawakens something in my heart.'

Bob is part of HelpForce, a charity started in 2017 to help patients and to support doctors and nurses. He works three mornings a week, helping the nurses organise the cutlery and food, visiting patients and trying to put them at ease. 'Some patients remember me when they come in again. I think, goodness, why do you remember *me*? Sometimes they say it's made their day to see my smiling face, and that's great.'

Bob is eager to tell me about the charity and his ideas for how to improve it. He takes this job as seriously as any paid role. 'I feel very strongly that staff must know they can count on the volunteers,' he says earnestly. 'My wife thinks volunteering is commendable, but that you can turn up when you want to. But if you don't come regularly, and come when you say you will, how can the staff rely on you?' For a mild-mannered, self-effacing man, he looks positively firm.

No job is too small. When someone is discharged, Bob will make the bed if the nurses are too busy: 'I'm on my feet the whole time. Sometimes I stay longer than the four hours, there's so much to be done. And the nurses work a 12-hour shift.'

Having run his own business, he can also stand back from the rush and look at the whole operation. 'I like the cleaners,' he says enthusiastically. 'They're a bit underrated, I think, and I try to encourage them.' A former designer, he feels it's important to try to make the spaces as habitable as possible. 'I think people react more positively to a space that is not in disarray so I'll pick litter off the floor, rearrange the chairs, put the monitors back to zero in the cubicles once patients have left. That's what I'd do at home.'

The word 'volunteering' can sound a bit weak. People often think of dutiful ladies working behind the counter in charity shops, or arranging flowers in a church. While there's nothing wrong with either of those, it is less well understood that dedicated volunteers can also make a real, measurable difference to public services. Since a HelpForce volunteer started calling people to remind them to go to their appointments at the memory clinic, attendance has leapt from 15 to 100 per cent. Others are driving patients to appointments, sitting with them through the consultation and taking notes, then dropping them home, sometimes picking up a pint of milk on the way. This is comforting, practical help for people who live alone, and a cost-saver for hospitals like this, whose annual bill for transporting patients home runs into the millions of pounds.

It is also a move back towards the original vision of the social reformer William Beveridge, of a shared project between the state and citizens. In 1942, Beveridge published what became the blueprint for the post-war UK welfare state. 'The state,' he wrote, 'in organising security, should not stifle incentive, opportunity, responsibility; in establishing a national minimum, it should leave room and encouragement for voluntary action by each individual to provide more than that minimum for himself and his family.'[13]

HelpForce is the brainchild of Tom Hughes-Hallett, former CEO of Marie Curie, the cancer charity, and now chair of London's Chelsea and Westminster Hospital. Hughes-Hallett is an awesomely lanky and irrepressible character with a booming voice and sharp eyes behind horn-rimmed glasses. What he is trying to do, he explains, is get back to Beveridge's principles, to 'the original NHS vision of shared benefit and shared responsibility'. And I rather think he will succeed.

'Today, we as citizens expect everything free in return for paying our taxes,' he continues. 'We have moved from a society that balanced rights and duties to a society that believes in duty-less rights. Unsurprisingly, compassionate communities have become a threatened species.'

By encouraging people to volunteer, Hughes-Hallett believes, he can relieve hard-pressed staff of basic burdens while giving patients more support. 'We are on a mission to inspire as many people as possible to enjoy being part of the health and care of British people,' he says. 'I would like to see volunteers underpinning every aspect of our NHS, which is to my mind the world's greatest health system.'

The benefits to the NHS are clear. But in Bob Groves' case, they are very much two-way. Before he became a volunteer, Bob confides, he suffered years of serious depression and anxiety, which damaged his relationship with his children. It's a huge shadow in his life that he feels he made a poor father. What do they think about him now? 'My children are admiring of me doing this,' he says proudly. Then he shrugs, sheepishly. 'I'm trying to get back into the world of normalcy, whatever that is. And no therapy has been as effective as volunteering.'

Second Acts for the Greater Good

In 2016, the *Financial Times* columnist Lucy Kellaway decided to break away from her prestigious, comfortable 31-year career in journalism, and launch into something totally different: teaching maths. With the social entrepreneur Katie Waldegrave she set up Now Teach, which recruits successful older people into full-time teaching. The two believed that those who had succeeded in other walks of life would have much to offer in the classroom. Of 35,000 trainee teachers in the UK, only 100 were over 55, despite the fact that there were serious teacher shortages in maths, science and languages, which many older people are good at.

The project has so far trained 120 teachers, who seem not to mind starting over at the bottom. Kellaway, 58, recently wrote that she had expected her social status to decline once she switched from journalism to teaching. In fact, she says, the opposite has happened. People seem admiring, and more interested, than before. 'Becoming a teacher in your 50s,' she has written, 'especially when you've had a certain amount of success doing something else, seems to be quite different from becoming one in your 20s.' Kellaway quoted a documentary-maker turned English teacher who felt the same. 'I think when we are young we imagine status comes from the outside,' this new teacher said. 'The approval, the promotion, the competition – all account for a "rise", as it were, as viewed from the outside. Now I am ancient, I realise that my ideas about status come much more from the inside. My own ideas about my contribution, my worth, are what count as status.'

Research supports this sense that, as we grow older, we become more interested in giving back. One study which tracked people over 50 years[14] found that they generally became warmer as they aged. The psychoanalyst Erik Erikson called this 'generativity': an impulse in older people to 'pass the torch' and help the next generation. According to the Stanford psychology professor Laura Carstensen, we tend to strive and fight when we are young, and the end of life seems far off. But as we grow older, we become more focused on meaningful experiences and close relationships. That may fill a deep need. George Vaillant, the Harvard psychiatrist quoted in Chapter 7, found that people in their seventies who mentored or supported others were three times happier, and had stronger marriages, than those who didn't.

Empower Success Corps, US

Ron Morin, 73, says he feels 'years younger' since having gone back to work, two decades after taking early retirement. Ron had given up his job at the age of 50 in order to paint and write. His wife ran a business, they have no children and they were financially comfortable. But 20 years later, things had not worked out quite as he'd hoped. His novels hadn't been published, though he'd had some successful local shows of his paintings. A play he wrote didn't make the big time, although it was produced by a local community group. 'I was moping around,' he says, 'not exactly sorry for myself but not feeling super-excited either.'

He started applying for jobs, but couldn't get an interview: 'I wasn't even looked at, I was sure it was because of my age.' Although he did not state his age on his CV, 'they would have been able to tell by my experience that I'd been around the block a couple of times'.

'You're kind of wasting away,' his wife told him. 'Why don't you volunteer? You'll feel better about yourself.'

Ron applied to Empower Success Corps, which pairs retired professionals with non-profit organisations in the U.S. He is now executive director of Friends of the Middlesex Fells, which manages a 3,000-acre forest in northern Massachusetts. It's the second largest urban forest in the world, and on the register of historic national sites: 'right up there with Mount Rushmore!' he chuckles.

'We have 183 bird species, 10 state-listed rare species of plant and 560 native plants which – by the way – are endangered. I've found out all sorts of things I didn't know before,' he says excitedly.

The Fells had younger applicants for the job, but they didn't have the managerial skills the board needed. 'What I had going for me was that I was a manager, I had restructured an organisation before and made it grow. A major weakness was that I am not a professional conservationist. But I know how to get the best out of people.'

Thousands more like Ron have found roles through ESC and its parent organisation, Encore.org, whose wonderful slogan is 'Second acts for the greater good'. Non-profits pay a finders' fee to ESC, which vets retired applicants carefully and trains them in governance and finance.

'It makes me feel good to help them,' Ron says. 'I'm using my brain. It's really good for me to solve problems, I'm dealing with politically difficult situations, finding solutions.' He imagines himself doing this 'as long as my health holds up. I want to create a Nature Centre, that will take a number of years to do as we will have to fundraise and design a building. I would love to do that for them. I would really like, at this time of life, to save a forest.'

Being Yourself

Every time I interview a volunteer, I ask what their friends think about it. Most say their friends admire them, but are not interested. 'They don't want that kind of responsibility any more,' one told me. 'They can see I've got more energy, they say I look better – but they don't want to get involved.' Not everyone is jumping to be a do-gooder, it seems.

I understand this. All his life, my father was absolutely resistant to joining any kind of club. He was hugely gregarious, and very kind, but had a complete aversion to the demands of any institution. He'd hated school and loathed his various office jobs. He found enormous enjoyment in being the quizmaster at his local church pub quiz night (my eternal thanks go to the vicar who dreamed that up). That role worked because it fitted who he was, and what he was good at. But there was no way I could persuade him to take tea to an elderly stranger, or join a group of over-80s on an outing. His important characteristic was not that he was in his eighties but that he was a writer and historian who loved jazz and cats – his age had nothing to do with who he was.

This point was brought home to me at a very upscale nursing home, Brookhaven, in Lexington, Massachusetts. I had gone there to visit the grandparents of one of the students at Harvard's Kennedy School. They were a wonderful couple, very attentive to each other and squeezing every moment out of life. He was a surgeon and still hearty, but she was frail and they had thought it wise to move while they still could. They were telling me about the new friends they'd made, and how he enjoyed helping to run the residents' grocery store, when she said to me reflectively: 'There aren't many other doctors here, though.' 'Oh,' he laughed, 'they're all up at X' (he named another home further north). He turned to me, smiling: 'We're

all Democrats here, you see. Up there, they're a bunch of Republicans.'
No one was going to rob him of his identity.

For me, this conversation echoed the legendary work done in one
nursing home by the psychologists Ellen Langer and Judith Rodin.
The residents were each given a houseplant for their room. Half were
told a nurse would look after it, the other half were told they were
responsible for it. The improvements in mental and physical wellbeing of the second group were so considerable that, 18 months later,
they were only half as likely as the first group to have died. It is an
excellent example of the importance of autonomy and identity to our
deepest selves.

Purpose Provides Structure

Few will thrive on 30 years of leisure. Some people are burned out;
others have caring responsibilities. But we have to wean ourselves off
this idea of the 'Golden Years' of leisure and regain our idealism
about what older people can offer, at a time when there are so many
societal problems to fix.

We need to see Extra Time as a starting point, not as the beginning
of the end. That might mean older people training younger ones on
the job; running preventative health programmes; acting as trusted
brokers in the care sector; or becoming teachers, social workers,
nurses: why not?

'When you run a marathon, at a certain point you hit the wall',
says Paul Irving, Chairman of the US Milken Institute Center for the
Future of Aging. 'Then you go through it. Towards the end, you get
the "kick". The fewer years we have left, the closer the end, the value
of our time goes up. We should see this as an opportunity to speed
up. We have to make people believe that this can be the most valuable time of their life.'

There could be few better statements of the fact that in Extra
Time, there is everything to play for.

10

Generation Hexed

We need a new social contract

FOR THE PAST 50 years, citizens growing up in industrialised countries have enjoyed an implicit social contract: work hard and pay tax, and you can expect rising living standards, a safety net if things go wrong and a pension. That contract is a powerful expression of social solidarity, one of the greatest achievements of the twentieth century. But it is now under threat.

Earlier in this book, we saw how the population pyramid, in which a wide band of young taxpayers traditionally supported a narrower group of older retirees, has fattened out (see pages 11–13). It's now shaped more like a barrel. As baby boomers retire, the number of beneficiaries keeps rising, relative to the number of taxpayers.[1] In 1950, globally, there were about 12 workers for every pensioner. Today, there are fewer than six in most developed countries and three in some parts of Europe. Unless pensioners start to work longer, current 'pay as you go' welfare systems will be unsustainable.

That's not all. In many countries a rising share of wealth and public spending is going to baby boomers (those born 1946–1965), less to generation X (those born 1965–1981) and less to millennials (those born 1981–1996). In the US, in Japan and in Europe, I have met people in their twenties and thirties who say they don't expect pensions to exist by the time they grow old. Some fear they will be worse-off than their parents. More and more, as we have seen, are putting off having children.

The social contract is being stretched to breaking point by the changing ratio of old to young, the increasing share of wealth owned by older generations and poor job prospects for the young. Yet despite pensioner poverty having been largely vanquished in most high-income countries, not all pensioners are well-off. The UK Centre for Ageing Better calculates that 12 per cent of over-65s are 'Struggling and Alone': socially isolated, poor and in bad health. While I believe passionately that we could improve lives by slashing the incidence of lifestyle diseases like type 2 diabetes – and save billions on healthcare – this will not happen overnight.

The big question is this: how can we provide a civilised old age without bankrupting the young?

It's not helpful, in my view, to stoke a war between millennials and baby boomers. The *New York Times* columnist Thomas L. Friedman has gloriously railed against 'a grasshopper generation, eating through just about everything like hungry locusts'. David Willetts, chair of the UK Resolution Foundation, has argued that 'the baby boomers took their children's future'. But it's not quite that simple, for two reasons. First, the generations are becoming more, not less, interdependent. The Bank of Mum and Dad is working overtime, and surveys suggest millennials don't especially support cutting elderly benefits.[2] Second, the new divide is not only between old and young, but between the networked, professional classes and the rest.

The New Divide: Unskilled v Skilled, Not Just Old v Young

The UK Brexit vote of 2016 was widely portrayed as a generational clash, with MP Vince Cable (aged 74), claiming, 'The older generation have shafted the young'. And indeed, less than a third of 18- to 24-year-olds voted to leave the EU, compared with two-thirds of over-65s. But the even bigger gap was between university graduates, who mostly voted to remain in the EU, and those with fewer qualifications, who overwhelmingly voted to leave.[3] As middling jobs are automated, the less skilled of all ages face a greater struggle to find stable, permanent work. This, in my view, is a divide which deserves just as much attention as that between the generations.

The well-meaning Bank of Mum and Dad is exacerbating this divide, by entrenching home ownership as an increasingly hereditary trait. One in four housing transactions in the UK is now eased along by financial contributions from parents.[4] Some parents may be over-reaching in their generosity – by taking money out of their pensions to help their children, when they themselves may still have decades to live. As the *Financial Times* columnist Merryn Somerset Webb has shrewdly observed, 'one of the greatest gifts a parent can give a child is their own financial security'.[4] But the upshot is generally to concentrate property wealth, the single most important asset that most people will ever own. Eighty-three per cent of millennials who own their own home have parents who do so too.[5] That's a problem.

The Plight of the Young

In 2005 I presented a programme for BBC Radio 4 entitled *Generation Hexed*, a title the editor and I were rather pleased with. The programme was about how the generation born in the 1970s and 1980s was finding it increasingly difficult to buy their own homes, was burdened with student debt and largely shut out of the generous company pension schemes enjoyed by those born in the post-war baby-boom years, many of whom were looking forward to an early and affluent retirement. Most of the millennials we interviewed were resigned, as I myself was, to the fact that they would never enjoy those kind of de luxe pensions. They expected to be relatively self-reliant, and prepared for the likelihood that they would need to work longer.

That was before the financial crisis of 2007–08.

Today's twenty- and thirty-somethings bore the brunt of the financial crisis. While wages are beginning to tick up again after the long drought, youth unemployment remains high in many European countries, sparking concerns about a lost generation. Insecurity is rife as automation wipes out many secure, mid-level jobs and self-employment is on the rise. Pay growth has been sluggish since the financial crisis and the swell of entry into universities has resulted in student debt, but not necessarily higher incomes.

The wealth gap between young and old has reached unprecedented levels for modern times. In the UK, millennial families are only half as likely to own their home by age 30 as baby boomers were by the same age[6]. They spend almost a quarter of their income on housing, compared to just 8 per cent spent by the Silent Generation (born 1929–46) at the same age. In 1983, the typical American older household was around eight times wealthier than the typical younger household. By 2013, it was 20 times wealthier.[7]

Baby boomers struggled to earn deposits and to pay high mortgage rates. But many also enjoyed the fruits of the inflating property bubble. Some younger people who did manage to get on the ladder experienced the full force of that bubble bursting.

There has been a fundamental shift in incomes too. In the UK, average pensioner household incomes are now greater than average working-age household incomes, after accounting for housing costs.[8] To add insult to injury, many high-income governments have borrowed billions, which the young will have to repay. In the UK, national debt currently stands at 84 per cent of GDP.[9] Taken together, this means that many rich countries are now at a point when 'an unprecedented claim on economic resources by the oldest generation' is said to be 'threatening the social contract between the generations and prospects for continued economic growth'. Those words come not from firebrand activists, politicians or self-hating baby-boomer columnists. They were written by two demure, respected demographers called Andrew Mason and Ronald Lee.

Professors Lee and Mason dig deep into the ways that demographic change distorts the altruistic impulse of humans to support both young and old. They have constructed a set of National Transfer Accounts which analyse in detail the flows of income, assets, savings and consumption in more than 60 countries around the world.[10] Throughout history, transfers have flowed downwards, from old to young. But population ageing has led to a steady decrease in the strength of this downward pattern.

In Japan, Germany, Austria, Slovenia and Hungary, rich nations with some of the oldest populations, Lee and Mason find that the direction of transfers has been *reversed*, probably for the first time in history. This means that current generations are now claiming the resources of future generations. If nothing is done, Lee and Mason predict that the direction of transfer flows will be reversed in many more countries by 2050. They cite two main reasons: age at retirement has declined and spending on healthcare has increased.[11]

This is no one's fault. It's a consequence of demography, and our failure to update our systems in response. But nor is it fair. For it suggests the young will be paying taxes to support a level of benefits for the old which they themselves may have no hope of receiving.

Politicians are understandably reluctant to break promises to older generations. They also hesitate to upset the grey vote. Many people who have worked hard and paid taxes believe they are entitled to 'take out' what they've 'paid in'. Unfortunately, it's not quite that simple. In pay-as-you-go welfare systems, today's workers don't put their taxes into a pot labelled with their name, waiting to be retrieved when they need it. Their taxes are paying the benefits of today's retirees. UK national insurance contributions and US payroll taxes are invested in government bonds, whose value depends on the ability of future taxpayers to service them.

The problem is that baby boomers are set to take out considerably more than they ever paid in, partly by just living longer. That is a key consequence of longevity: welfare systems which were designed to redistribute wealth from rich to poor, from healthy to disabled and from young to old are now redistributing wealth from everyone – to those who live longer. And those who live longest are likely to be those who are wealthiest.

The Plight of the Old

One of my favourite film sequences in recent years is the shoplifting scene in *Going in Style*, the 2017 film starring Morgan Freeman and Michael Caine. The two pensioners, down on their luck, plot to steal groceries from their local supermarket. Freeman sneaks down the aisles and bags the loot. The moment when Caine picks him up in the get away vehicle, which turns out to be an electric mobility scooter, is a classic of modern cinema.

When I visited Japan, I was surprised to find that such scenes are no longer fiction. The country has been hit by a crime wave of elderly shoplifters. A staggering 20 per cent of the entire Japanese prison population is now aged over 60 (compared to 6 per cent in the US).[12] And unlike the fictitious characters played by Freeman and Caine, these thieves seem to want to be caught – because they can't make ends meet.

'What we are seeing is a deliberate attempt to break into prison as a way to survive,' says Michael Newman, who runs a consulting firm, Custom Products Research, out of Tokyo. Newman, an ebullient New Zealander who looks like a rugby forward but is actually a statistics nerd, discovered that a strange spike in elderly crime was being caused by pensioners on meagre incomes who were repeatedly re-offending.[13]

These are the forgotten people: men with no savings and widows of salarymen whose pensions did not automatically transfer to their wives. Traditionally, they would have been looked after by relatives, but a 2017 survey by the Japanese government found that over half of elderly shoplifters lived alone.[14] In prison, Newman points out, 'they get a roof over their head, three square meals a day, no utility bills and unlimited free healthcare'.

One prison inmate, a Ms F, 89, told a Bloomberg reporter that she had stolen rice, strawberries and cold medicine. 'I was living alone on welfare,' she said. 'I used to live with my daughter's family and used all my savings taking care of an abusive and violent son-in-law.'[15]

This influx of unlikely criminals is turning Japan's prisons into old-age care homes. Specialised staff have been hired to help elderly people with dressing and washing. Prison medical bills have jumped by 80 per cent in ten years.[16]

Michael Newman thinks it would be cheaper, and more humane, for the government to build large-scale dormitories, where poor elderly folk could trade in their pensions for food and medical facilities. They could do this, he thinks, on the vast tracts of land which are emptying out as youngsters seek their fortunes in the cities. In ten years' time, this might become an attractive solution.

I tell this story because it highlights a hidden seam of persistent poverty which plagues many countries. In the UK, 1.9 million pensioners are living on less than 60 per cent of median national income (median national income is £28,400 a year).[17] In the US, it is estimated that as many as 40 per cent of middle-class pensioners could fall into poverty.[18] Large numbers of baby boomers haven't saved enough for retirement, foolishly or not, partly because they underestimated how long they might have to live. Low interest rates have hurt the savings of pensioners on fixed incomes, while boosting younger borrowers with mortgages. Moreover, personal pensions have become far less secure, for those who have them at all, with 'defined benefit' schemes, which used to guarantee an annual fixed income, being overtaken by volatile 'defined contribution' schemes which depend on market fluctuations. Responsibility for savings has been pushed from employers to workers in all but the most cosseted parts of the public sector. Larry Fink, chairman of the world's biggest money manager Blackrock, cited this shift as 'an underappreciated driver of popular anxiety' in his 2017 letter to shareholders.

Modern personal pensions are, frankly, mad. Even the most astute accountant must find it hard to plan for retirement when they don't know (a) how long they will live, (b) whether they may become too ill to work, (c) what the inflation rate will be. Employers have understandably retreated from taking on open-ended risk, as people live longer. But we have swung too far in the other direction. A better system would split the risk between employers and employees, and link pension ages to life expectancy.

For the most part the baby boomers are still much better off than the millennials, especially if they own their house. But as we redraw social safety nets, it is vital not to lose sight of the groups who are still in need.

Not Everything That Counts Is Being Counted

One piece missing from the argument about intergenerational unfairness is the fact that longer lives and financial strains are turning the baby boomers into the new 'sandwich' generation: more likely to be caring for elderly parents, supporting adult children or caring for grandchildren than any cohort before them.

Australian grandparents clock up an average of 58 childcare hours per month, equivalent to around $328 million in childcare every month.[19] In Italy and Portugal, around one grandmother in five provides daily care for a grandchild,[20] freeing up parents to go out to work. In the US, nearly a quarter of pre-school children are cared for by a grandparent, and one in ten lives in a household headed by a grandparent.[21] British grandparents save parents almost £2,000 a year in childcare fees,[22] and unpaid older caregivers in Britain save the state around £11.4 billion per year.[23]

Then there's community work. Older Americans spent 3.3 billion hours volunteering in 2016, the equivalent of an economic contribution worth $78 billion.[24] Shouldn't that appear somewhere on the balance sheet?

One answer, from three demographers in Denmark and Hungary – Pieter Vanhysse, Robert Gal and Lili Vargha – has been to value all of the cash and time given by older people in the UK, France, Germany, Italy, Spain, Finland and Sweden. They have tried to quantify everything from childcare to gardening. When all of these 'family transfers' are included, they argue that childhood – the period of being in receipt – now extends to 25, and independent adulthood – the period of making net contributions – lasts until 79. On that basis, they argue that while the old receive more from the state, the young get more from society: 'Europe is a continent of pro-elderly welfare states, embedded within societies composed of strongly child-oriented families.'[25]

These calculations can be criticised, not least because they define contribution so broadly. But they make the point that public money is not the only thing that matters: family matters too. The family is arguably responding more nimbly than governments.

Rewriting the Social Contract

It will soon become impossible for governments to keep all the promises made to the old without eating up a disproportionate share of the pie. Already, pension funds are failing and some local government schemes are bankrupt. Moreover, the divergence in life expectancy means that richer and more educated people are likely to live longer, earn more and receive more from welfare systems than anyone ever intended.

A basic principle must surely be that no generation should be asked to provide a higher level of support for the older generation than it can expect to receive. The obvious starting point is to challenge the institutional concept that old age starts at 65 and the practice – in many Western countries – of retiring even earlier. As we saw in Chapter 2, this no longer makes sense when life expectancy has risen so much. In Switzerland, France, Germany and Austria, over a third of over-65s say they are open to keep working: far more than are actually in the workforce at the moment.[26] It will be vital to help those people find jobs.

The challenge in the UK was exacerbated by the 2011 decision to protect pensions through a 'triple-lock', which indexed pensions to whichever was higher: the rate of inflation, wage rises, or 2.5 per cent. Weak earnings growth and low inflation resulted in pensions rising at twice the rate of worker wages.[27] That is neither fair nor sustainable. It would make sense to remove the 2.5 per cent element of the triple-lock, raise pension ages in line with life expectancy, and remove the anomaly whereby people who work past state pension age are exempt from the national insurance tax paid by all other workers on their earnings.

Protests in Greece and France have shown just how difficult it is for governments to remove entitlements. Public policy usually works best when everyone trades something for a collective gain. That was what Germany and Japan achieved in creating their social care insurance schemes. In the UK, such a scheme could be part-funded by removing the national insurance anomaly, which could raise almost £1 billion a year.[28] That might win public support, if it achieved a secure safety net for old age.

Challenging Fatalism

We can't keep putting off the day of reckoning. The generation which is now turning 65 will derive far more benefit from the welfare state than it will contribute in taxes. Unless we act, younger generations will pay the price. Yet this need not be a counsel of despair, if we challenge the fatalism which surrounds ageing. The 'demographic time bomb' scenarios assume that productivity declines after 50; that people continue to retire at 65 or earlier; that more and more people fall sick with chronic diseases; and that we are on a grim journey to spiralling health and welfare costs, with fewer people paying more and more taxes. But we are not, actually, 'ageing' as fast as the numbers suggest. In Extra Time, people can live longer, work longer, contribute longer than ever before. The challenge is to ensure that the 'Young-Old' can contribute productively to the economy, while the 'Old-Old' receive the support they need.

We must also support the family, the oldest safety net of all. That could mean paying relatives to be carers – something Germany is experimenting with. It should certainly mean providing respite periods for those who want to keep looking after their spouse but who are at breaking point. A comprehensive system of social care, funded through insurance, could transform what are currently fragmented, fear-inducing systems in the UK, US and other countries. If we are to move forward, however, we must ditch the stereotype of baby boomers bounding selfishly around the world on cruise ships, betraying the young. Demography is not a hostile act. Many in that generation are, in fact, doing a great deal for the young. We need to harness their energies to do even more.

An older man who joined one of my study groups at Harvard said wistfully to the students that he would like to find a way to contribute. 'There are so many challenges,' he said, reflectively. 'Climate change, poverty, housing. I feel we are all in this together. We older folk have more time: we should be using it. Tell us how to use it.' Extra Time is an opportunity to channel the altruism and energy of the 'Young-Old' into a better future for all.

Epilogue

A Different, Better World

FOR ME, THE ADVENT of Extra Time is one of the most dramatic stories of our age.

We are living through unprecedented demographic changes, which will have far-reaching global consequences. Shrinking populations will soon alter the balance of power between countries, and change the politics of immigration. Longevity is bringing back multi-generational households and creating age-diverse workforces. A dramatically changing ratio of older to younger people will force governments to rewrite the social contract, and to act against the junk-food merchants and fatalists who say that declining health is inevitable – when in fact the true biological path of ageing could look very different.

We are not ready. We are used to thinking of 'old' as 60, of early retirement as desirable, of dementia as inevitable, of good ideas and energy coming only from the 'young'. In fact, we don't like thinking about growing old at all, so we haven't noticed that 'old' is being redefined. We haven't even fully realised how long we might have to live – or planned for it.

Much of this should be good news. In the Fourth Industrial Revolution, we are consumed by fears that AI and robots will take our jobs. But the coming shortage of humans could tip economic power back from capital towards labour, as companies scrabble to find enough human talent. If we create a Fourth Stage of Education, we can rejuvenate and mobilise many people who are already 'unretiring' in pursuit of income, purpose and camaraderie. We can use their talents to help fix all sorts of societal problems.

We are equally prone to a fatalism about declining health. But there is now overwhelming evidence that healthier lifestyles, especially exercise, can be a miracle cure. We need to be much more ambitious for ourselves, and for our health systems, which must change from factories which were built to heal the sick, and send them on their way, into networks which help people stay independent and healthy as long as possible.

Government, businesses and the media can help, by changing the signals they send about age. New institutions will be needed: start-up trade unions to help people navigate the gig economy, multiversities to keep people learning, community membership organisations which bring strangers together, co-housing co-operatives, nursing teams where humanity trumps bureaucracy; social care insurance schemes; new medical licensing models which treat ageing as a disease; and better ways of measuring and targeting healthy life expectancy. There are good ideas coming from many countries, if we only look.

I have tried to show in this book that there are numerous ways in which we can improve our own odds of enjoying whatever time we have left to us. But we all know that ageing remains a lottery. None of us can dictate our own ending, and none of us should blame others for theirs. We need, above all, to be kinder. Most of us are destined to grow old one day. If we do nothing else, it surely makes sense to follow the old maxim: 'Do as you would be done by.'

This book began with the story of the flamboyant Dutchman who wanted to become legally 20 years younger. He told his friends he didn't want to lie about his age. That, perhaps, should be our goal. If we can reach the point that none of us ever feel we have to lie about our age, we will have fully embraced Extra Time.

Endnotes

(All web addresses correct at the time of going to press.)

Introduction

1. Bingham, John, 'Queen's "birthday card team" expands to cope with surge of 100-year-olds', *Telegraph* Online, 25 September 2014.
2. 'Life expectancy and healthy life expectancy', *Health Profile for England*, Public Health England, 2017.
3. 'US life expectancy falls for third year in a row', *BMJ*, 2018, 363, k5118.
4. Chen, A., Munnell, A.H., Sanzenbacher, G.T., Zulkarnain, A., 'Why Has U.S. Life Expectancy Fallen Below Other Countries?' Boston College Center for Retirement Brief, December 2017, http://crr.bc.edu/wp-content/uploads/2017/11/IB_17-22.pdf.
5. 'The Cavendish Review: An Independent Review into Healthcare Assistants and Support Workers in the NHS and Social Care Settings', Department of Health, July 2013.
6. The Care Quality Commission.

1. The Death of Birth

1. US Census Bureau, 'An Aging World: 2015', March 2016.
2. United Nations Population Division, World Population Prospects: 2017 Revision.

3. Census reports, and other statistical publications from national statistical offices, taken from World Bank Group.

4. Ibid.

5. Ibid.

6. The UN projects world population of 8.6 billion in 2030, 9.8 billion in 2050 and 11.2 billion in 2100. The International Institute for Applied Systems Analysis (IIASA) forecasts world population will peak at 9.4 billion around 2070, then decline to around 9 billion by 2100.

7. Takenaka, Kiyoshi, 'Ageing Japan – Akita prefecture may be glimpse of country's greying future', Reuters Online, July 2018.

8. 'Law requires Chinese to visit their aging parents', *Yahoo News*, July 2, 2013.

9. Hatton, Celia, 'New China law says children "must visit parents",' BBC News Online, July 2013.

10. 'In rapidly aging Japan, adult diaper sales are about to surpass baby diapers', *The Atlantic*, July 2013.

11. 'In sexless Japan, almost half of single young men and women are virgins: survey', *Japan Times*, 2016.

12. 'Single living trend continues to grow in Japan', Nippon Online, April 2018.

13. *The Fifteenth Japanese National Fertility Survey, 2015*, National Institute of Population and Social Security Research.

14. National Bureau of Statistics, China.

15. 'China's population set to peak at 1.44 billion in 2029 – government report', Reuters, January 2019.

16. Wangshu, Luo, 'New rules for visas to help Chinese "return home"', *China Daily* Online, January 2017. Attracting Skilled International Migrants to China: A review and comparison of policies and practices, International Labour Organisation Report, 2017.

17. Xinying, Zhao, 'Authorities working on plan to delay retirements', *China Daily Online,* July 2017.

18. The World Bank Online Data Set, 'Life Expectancy at Birth (Total Years)'.

19. Wang Feng and Mason, Andrew, 'The demographic factor in China's transition', in Loren Brandt and Thomas G. Rawski, eds, *China's Great Economic Transformation* (Cambridge: Cambridge University Press, 2008), 136–66.

20. United Nations Population Division, World Population Prospects: 2017 Revision.

21. World Bank 2007.

22. Livingstone, Gretchen, 'Over the past 25 years, immigrant moms bolstered births in 48 states', Pew Research Analysis of National Center for Health Statistics Data, Pew Research Center.

23. Ibid.

24. 'US women are postponing motherhood, but not as much as other as in most other developed nations', *Pew Research Center Fact Tank,* June 2018.

25. Case, Anne and Deaton, Angus, 'Rising morbidity and mortality in midlife among white non-Hispanic Americans in the 21st century', *Proceedings of the National Academy of Sciences*, 2015, 1–6.

26. Centers for Disease Control and Prevention, 'Mortality in the United States 2016', US Department of Health and Human Services, https://www.cdc.gov/nchs/data/databriefs/db293.pdf.

27. Centers for Disease Control and Prevention.

28. 'The empty crib', *The Economist,* August 2016.

29. Jensen, Robert and Oster, Emily, 'The power of TV: cable television and women's status in India', *Quarterly Journal of Economics*, 2009, 124 (3), 1057–94.

30. La Ferrara, Eliana, Chong, Alberto and Duryea, Suzanne, 'Soap operas and fertility: evidence from Brazil', *American Economic Journal: Applied Economics*, 2012, 4 (4), 1–31.

31. Kotkin, Joel, 'Singapore's midlife crisis', *City Journal* Online, March 2016.

32. Population Trends 2017, Department of Statistics, Singapore.

33. Instituto Nazionale de Statistica.

34. European Commission/Eurostat, 'Mean age of women at childbirth across EU regions', Eurostat Data.

35. European Commission/Eurostat, 'Young people living with their parents', Eurostat Data.

36. Edwards, Catherine, 'The real reasons young Italians aren't having kids', *The Local, Italy,* September 2016.

37. Istat, 2011.

38. Reiter, Chris, 'How Germany is defusing a demographic time bomb', Bloomberg Online, May 2018.

39. HMG, *Public Expenditure: Statistical Analyses 2017*, Controller of Her Majesty's Stationery Office, 2017.

40. UK Office for National Statistics, 'Births by Parents' Country of Birth, England and Wales: 2017'.

41. UK Office for National Statistics, 'Births in England and Wales: 2017'.

42. 'Trends in life expectancy in EU and other OECD countries: Why are improvements slowing?', OECD Health Working Paper 108, Veena S. Raleigh (The King's Fund), 28 Feb 2019

43. 'Great Expectations', *RBC Capital Markets*, 13 February, 2019

44. United Nations Population Division, World Population Prospects: 2017 Revision. There are differing projections as to world population growth. The UN projects world population of 8.6 billion in 2030, 9.8 billion in 2050 and 11.2 billion in 2100 (https://www.un.org/development/desa/en/news/population/world-population-prospects-2017.html). However, the International Institute for Applied Systems Analysis (IIASA) forecasts world population will peak at 9.4 billion around 2070, then decline to around 9 billion by 2100, (http://www.iiasa.ac.at/web/home/about/news/20141023-population-9billion.html). The new UN paper uses a probabilistic approach to global population projections providing quantitative uncertainty ranges. The IIASA, however, were based on 'input of more than 550 experts worldwide who were invited to evaluate in a peer review manner a set of alternative scientific arguments bearing directly on the future demographic trajectories'. The IIASA give greater weight to the importance of education levels and consequent decline of fertility rates and population growth. Geographically, most of the discrepancy in the

projections relates to Africa, given differing assumptions about future fertility. A fuller explanation of the difference between the two projections is detailed in an IIASA Research Blog (https://blog.iiasa.ac.at/2014/09/23/9-billion-or-11-billion-the-research-behind-new-population-projections/) and an analysis by the Brookings Institution (https://www.brookings.edu/blog/future-development/2015/09/04/will-the-world-reach-10-billion-people/).

45. 'Tanzania's President Magufuli calls for end to birth control', BBC News Online, September 2018.

46. Davis VanOpdorp, 'Polish government urges citizens to multiply like rabbits', *DW.com*, 8 November 2017.

2. Younger Than You Thought

1. 'Scientists up stakes in bet on whether humans will live to 150', *Nature*, October 2016.

2. Sawyer, S., et al, 'The age of adolescence', *Lancet Child and Adolescent Health*, 2018, 2 (3), 223–8.

3. Jagger, C., Matthews, F.E., et al., 'A comparison of health expectancies over two decades in England: results of the Cognitive Function and Ageing Study I and II', *Lancet*, 2016, 387: 779–86.

4. 'The Population 65 Years and Older in the United States: 2016', American Community Survey Reports, October 2018.

5. YouGov Poll, 'Are you worried about dementia?', May 2012.

6. NHS dementia guide.

7. Qiu, C., von Strauss, E., Bäckman, L., Winblad, B., Fratiglioni, L., 'Twenty-year changes in dementia occurrence suggest decreasing incidence in central Stockholm, Sweden', *Neurology*, 2013, 80, 1888–94.

8. Ahmadi-Abhari, S., Guzman-Castillo, M., et al., 'Temporal trend in dementia incidence since 2002 and projections for prevalence in England and Wales to 2040: modelling study', *BMJ*, 2017, 358, j2856. Matthews, F.E., Stephan, B., et al., 'A two-decade dementia incidence comparison from the Cognitive Function and Ageing Studies I and II', *Nature Communications*, 2016, 7 (11398).

9. Kolata, Gina, 'U.S. dementia rates are dropping even as population ages', *New York Times* Online, November 2016.

10. Satizabal, C.L., Beiser, A. Chouraki, V., Chêne, G., Dufouil, C., Seshadri, S., 'Incidence of dementia over three decades in the Framingham Heart Study', *New England Journal of Medicine*, 2016, 374, 523–32.

11. The German retirement age is now 65 for people born before 1947, and 67 for those born after 1964.

12. 'Economic labour market status of individuals aged 50 and over, trends over time', Department of Work and Pensions, October 2018.

13. UK Office for National Statistics, 'How has life expectancy changed over time?', September 2009.

14. UK Office for National Statistics, National Life Tables, UK: 2015 to 2017.

15. Sanderson, W.C. and Scherbov, S., 'Faster increases in human life expectancy could lead to slower population aging', *PLoS One*, 2015, 10 (4), e0121922.

16. 'Fifty-somethings should be forced to work until 70', *Daily Telegraph*, 20 May 2016.

17. Normand, Patrice, 'How to be sexy at 50 (according to French dating expert Mylène Desclaux)', *The Times* Online, 24 November 2018.

18. Cavendish, Camilla, 'The Magazine Interview: Margaret Atwood, author of *The Handmaid's Tale*', *Sunday Times Magazine*, 29 October 2017.

19. Matthews, Steve, 'Here's proof that age discrimination is widespread in the job market', Bloomberg Online, October 2015.

20. Levy, Becca, 'Stereotype embodiment: a psychosocial approach to aging', *Current Directions in Psychological Science*, 2009, 18 (6), 332–6.

21. 'Jerry Hayes: Treasury cuts have crippled justice system', *The Times*, 15 December 2017.

22. Olshanksy, S.J., Antonucci, T., et al., 'Differences in life expectancy due to race and educational differences are widening, and many may not catch up', *Health Affairs*, 2012, 31 (8), 1803–13.

23. 'Life expectancy by sex and education level', Health at a Glance, OECD Indicators.

24. Mackenzie, Debora, 'More education is what makes people live longer, not more money', *New Scientist*, April 2018.

25. Office for National Statistics, Life Expectancy at Birth, Westminster Council Ward Profiles.

26. Jagger, Carol, 'We need a completely new approach to caring for people', *Independent*, 20 October 2014.

27. J House et al, 'Continuity and Change in the Social Stratification of Aging and Health Over the Life Course' *The Journals of Gerontology: Series B*, Volume 60, Issue Special Issue_2, 1 October 2005, Pages S15–S26.

28. Marmot, M. and Brunner, E., 'Cohort profile: the Whitehall II study', *International Journal of Epidemiology*, 2005, 34 (2), 251–6.

29. Kuper, H. and Marmot, M., 'Job strain, job demands, decision latitude, and risk of coronary heart disease within the Whitehall II study', *Journal of Epidemiology and Community Health*, 2003, 57 (2), 147–53.

30. Jagger, C., 'Trends in life expectancy and healthy life expectancy', Newcastle Institute for Ageing, 2015.

31. Ministerial Notification No. 430, Ministry of Health, Labour and Welfare, Japan.

32. Comprehensive Survey of Living Conditions, Ministry of Health, Labour and Welfare, Japan.

33. Japan Ministry of Labour, Health and Welfare, Abridged Life Tables for Japan, 2013 and 2016.

34. www.springchicken.co.uk.

3. Just Do It

1. McPhee, J.S., French, D.P., et al., 'Physical activity in older age: perspectives for healthy ageing and frailty', *Biogerontology*, 2016, 17 (3), 567–80. Daskalopoulou, C., Stubbs, B., et al., 'Physical activity and healthy ageing: a systematic review and meta-analysis of longitudinal cohort studies', *Ageing Research Reviews*, 2017, 38, 6–17.

2. Academy of Medical Royal Colleges, 'Exercise – the Miracle Cure', 2015.

3. Pollock, R.D., et al., 'Properties of the vastus lateralis muscle in relation to age and physiological function in master cyclists aged 55–79 years', *Aging Cell*, 2018, e12735.

4. Buettner, Dan, *The Blue Zones* (Boone, IA: National Geographic Books, 2008).

5. Gries, K.J., et al., 'Cardiovascular and skeletal muscle health with lifelong exercise', *Journal of Applied Physiology*, 2018, 125 (5), 1636–45.

6. Akkari, A., Machin, D., Tanaka, H., 'Greater progression of athletic performance in older Masters athletes', *Age and Ageing*, 2015, 44 (4), 683–6.

7. Reaburn, P. and Dascombe, B., 'Endurance performance in masters athletes', *European Review of Aging and Physical Activity*, 2008, 5, 29.

8. 'Olympian lifespan possible for all', BBC News Online, 14 December 2012.

9. Curtis, E., Litwic, A., Cooper, C., Dennison, E., 'Determinants of muscle and bone aging', *Journal of Cell Physiology*, 2015, 230 (11), 2618–25.

10. 'Physical activity 2016: progress and challenges', *Lancet* Series.

11. Morris, J.N., Heady, J.A., Raffle, P.A., Roberts, C.G., Parks, J.W., 'Coronary heart-disease and physical activity of work', *Lancet*, 1953, 265, 1111–20.

12. Bey, L. and Hamilton, M.T., 'Suppression of skeletal muscle lipoprotein lipase activity during physical inactivity: a molecular reason to maintain daily low-intensity activity', *Journal of Physiology*, 2003, 551 (Pt 2), 673–82.

13. Lee, I.M. and Skerrett, P.J., 'Physical activity and all-cause mortality: what is the dose–response relation?', *Medicine & Science in Sports and Exercise*, 2011, 33 (6 Suppl), S459–71.

14. Tigbe, W.W., et al., 'Time spent in sedentary posture is associated with waist circumference and cardiovascular risk', *International Journal of Obesity*, 2017, 41, 689–96.

15. McNally, S., Nunan, D., Dixon, A., Maruthappu, M., Butler, K., Gray, M., et al., 'Focus on physical activity can help avoid unnecessary social care', *BMJ*, 2017, 359, j4609.

16. Cadore, Eduardo, Casas, Alvaro, et al., 'Multicomponent exercises including muscle power training enhance muscle mass, power output, and functional outcomes in institutionalized frail nonagenarians', *Age (Dordrecht, Netherlands)*, 2014, 36 (2), 773–85.

17. Age UK, 'Falls Prevention Exercise – following the evidence', 2013.

18. 'Exercise for Life: Physical Activity in Health and Disease', Royal College of Physicians Working Paper, 2012.

19. Gillespie, L.D., Robertson, M.C., Gillespie, W.J., Sherrington, C., Gates, S., Clemson, L.M., Lamb, S.E., 'Interventions for preventing falls in older people living in the community', *Cochrane Database of Systematic Reviews*, 2012, 9, Art. No.CD007146.

20. Stanmore et al., 'The effectiveness and cost-effectiveness of strength and balance Exergames to reduce falls risk for people aged 55 years and older in UK assisted living facilities: a multi-centre, cluster randomised controlled trial', *BMC Medicine*, to be published 2019.

21. 'Making prescription drugs free for people 65 and over', Premier of Ontario, News Release.

22. 'Treatment to delay dementia by five years would reduce cases by 33%', Alzheimer's Research UK, June 2014.

23. Among men; women had a much lower risk, which is why women were not included in the study.

24. Elwood, Peter, et al., 'Healthy lifestyles reduce the incidence of chronic diseases and dementia: evidence from the Caerphilly cohort study', *PloS One*, 2013, 8 (12), e81877.

25. Mostly attributable to giving up smoking.

26. 'Prof. Peter Elwood on exercise link to avoiding dementia', BBC News Online Video.

27. Livingston, Gill, et al., 'Dementia prevention, intervention, and care', The Lancet Commission, *Lancet*, 2017, 390 (10113).

28. Cadore, Eduardo, Casas, Alvaro, et al., 'Multicomponent exercises including muscle power training enhance muscle mass, power output, and functional outcomes in institutionalized frail nonagenarians', *Age (Dordrecht, Netherlands)*, 2014, 36 (2), 773–85.

29. Livingston, Gill, et al., 'Dementia prevention, intervention, and care', The Lancet Commission, *Lancet*, 2017, 390 (10113).

30. Dr Sally Fenton, 'Why can't parents recognise when their children are overweight or obese?', University of Birmingham Online Blog.

31. OECD, *Health at a Glance 2017: OECD Indicators* (Paris: OECD Publishing, 2017).

32. US Centers for Disease Control.

33. 'Road cycling: statistics', House of Commons Library Standard Note: SN/SG/06224, 2013.

34. 'Study: surge in obesity correlates with increased automobile usage', *University of Illinois Online Research News Post*, https://news.illinois.edu/view/6367/205328.

35. Ronan, L., et al., 'Obesity associated with increased brain-age from mid-life', *Neurobiology of Aging*, 2016, 47, 63–70.

36. Diabetes UK, 'Number of people living with diabetes doubles in twenty years', Research Factsheet, https://www.diabetes.org.uk/about_us/news/diabetes-prevalence-statistics.

37. Corriere, M., et al., 'Epidemiology of diabetes and diabetes complications in the elderly: an emerging public health burden', *Current Diabetes Reports*, 2013, 13 (6), 805–13.

38. Lustig, Robert, *Fat Chance, The Hidden Truth About Sugar* (New York: Hudson Street Press, 2013).

39. Wansini, B. and Kim, J., 'Bad popcorn in big buckets: portion size can influence intake as much as taste', *Journal of Nutritional Educational Behaviour*, 2005, 37 (5): 242–5.

40. 'Sugar levy leaves bitter taste for drinks makers', *Financial Times*, 1 April 2018.

41. Aveyard, P., et al., 'Screening and brief intervention for obesity in primary care: a parallel, two-arm, randomised trial', *Lancet*, 2016, 388 (10059), 2492–500.

42. Booth, H.P., Prevost, T., Gulliford, M.C., 'Access to weight reduction interventions for overweight and obese patients in UK primary care: population-based cohort study', *BMJ Open*, 2015, 5 (1), e006642.

43. According to a 2010 study published in *Preventative Cardiology*, less than one-fifth of US attending physicians, and only 10 per cent of medical trainees, felt confident to bring up weight.

44. Lean, M. et al., 'Primary care-led weight management for remission of type 2 diabetes (DiRECT): an open-label, cluster-randomised trial', *Lancet*, 2018, 391 (10120), 541–51.

45. Jebb, S.A., Astbury, N.M., et al., 'Doctor Referral of Overweight People to a Low-Energy Treatment (DROPLET) in primary care using total diet replacement products: a protocol for a randomised controlled trial', *BMJ Open*, 2017, 7, e016709.

46. 'Severe obesity four times more likely in poor primary schools', BBC News, October 2018.

47. Andrea T. Feinberg, MD, Allison Hess, Michelle Passaretti, BSN, RN, CCM, Stacy Coolbaugh, MBA, RDN, LDN & Thomas H. Lee, MD, MSc, 'Prescribing Food as a Specialty Drug', 10 April 2018, Geisinger Health System, 10 April 2018.

48. OECD Indicators, 'Health at a Glance 2013'.

4. No Desire to Retire

1. Kashiwagi, Shigeo, 'Japan must abolish mandatory retirement', *Nikkei Asian Review* Online, May 2018.

2. Ibid.

3. Mankad, Prerna, 'Japan finds the cure for Retired Husband Syndrome', *Foreign Policy*, April 2007.

4. 'Spring cleaning: Japan's grey divorcees', *The Economist*, April 2016.

5. UK Office for National Statistics, 'Marriage and divorce on the rise at 65 and over', ONS Online Factsheet, July 2017.

6. Hill, Amelia, 'Older entrepreneurs employ more staff than start-ups run by younger people', *Guardian*, December 2017.

7. Kauffman Foundation, 'Startup Activity Reports', 2017.

8. Azoulay, Pierre, Jones, Benjamin, Kim, J. Daniel, Miranda, Javier, 'Research: the average age of a successful startup founder is 45', *Harvard Business Review*, July 2018, https://hbr.org/2018/07/research-the-average-age-of-a-successful-startup-founder-is-45.

9. 'Who pays the bill?', *The Economist*, July 20013, https://www.economist.com/united-states/2013/07/27/who-pays-the-bill.

10. McMahon, E.J. and McGee, Josh B., 'The never-ending hangover: how New York City's pension costs threaten its future', The Manhattan Institute, June 2017.

11. www.fidelity.com.

12. OECD Data Library, 'Pensions at a Glance 2011'.

13. PwC, 'Golden Age Index', June 2018.

14. OECD Data Set, 'Employment Rate by Age Group'.

15. PwC, 'Golden Age Index', June 2018.

16. Lee, Ronald and Mason, Andrew, *Population Aging and the Generational Economy: A Global Perspective* (Cheltenham: Edward Elgar, 2011).

17. Maestas, Nicole, 'Back to work: expectations and realizations of work after retirement', *Journal of Human Resources*, 2010, 45 (3), 718–48.

18. Davis, Kevin, 'The age of retirement', AIST-ACFS Research Project, 2013.

19. Maestas, Nicole, Mullen, Kathleen J., Powell, David, von Wachter, Till, Wenger, Jeffrey B., *Working Conditions in the United States: Results of the 2015 American Working Conditions Survey* (Santa Monica, CA: RAND Corporation, 2017).

20. Maestas, Nicole, Mullen, Kathleen J., Powell, David, von Wachter, Till, Wenger, Jeffrey B., *The American Working Conditions Survey Finds*

That More Than Half of Retirees Would Return to Work (Santa Monica, CA: RAND Corporation, 2017).

21. Schneider, Howard, 'INSIGHT – Many who have left U.S. labor force say they would like to return', Reuters, August 2014.

22. Ibid.

23. Drydakis, Nick, MacDonald, Peter, Chiotis, Vangelis, Somers, Laurence, 'Age discrimination in the UK labour market: does race moderate ageism? An experimental investigation', *Applied Economics Letters, 2018,* 25 (1), 1–4.

24. Neumark, David, Burn, Ian, Button, Patrick, 'Age Discrimination and Hiring of Older Workers', Research from the Federal Reserve Bank of San Francisco, February 2017.

25. 'Older workers failed by weak enforcement of age discrimination', Women and Equalities Select Committee Report, July 2018.

26. Court of Appeal, Fourth District, Division 1, California: George Corley, Plaintiff and Respondent, v. San Bernardino County Fire Protection District, Defendant and Appellant. D072852. Decided: 15 March 2018.

27. OECD Data Set, 'Employment Rate by Age Group'.

28. Munnell, Alicia and Wu, April Yanyuan, 'Will Delayed Retirement by the Baby Boomers Lead to Higher Unemployment Among Younger Workers?', Boston College Center for Retirement Research Working Paper No. 2012-22, September 2012.

29. Marangozov, Rachel, Williams, Matthew, Buchan, James, 'The labour market for nurses in the UK and its relationship to the demand for, and supply of, international nurses in the NHS', *Institute for Employment Studies,* July 2016.

30. UK Office for National Statistics, 'Agriculture in the United Kingdom 2017', Department for Environment, Food and Rural Affairs, 2018.

31. 'Where have the skilled workers gone?', *Der Spiegel,* 22 June 2007.

32. Wong, Perry, Chng, Belinda, Garcia, Amos, Burstein, Arielle, 'Redefining Traditional Notions of Aging', Milken Institute Center for the Future of Aging, 2016.

33. Yamamoto 2013, quoted in Sanzenbacher, Geoffrey and Sass, Steven, 'Is working longer a good prescription for all?' *Center for Retirement Research at Boston College, Issue in Brief*, 2017, 17–21.

34. 'Gender Pay Gap Service', Online Portal.

35. UK Office for National Statistics, UK Survey of Carers in Households – England, 2010.

36. Elkins, Kathleen, 'Here's the age at which you'll earn the most in your career', CNBC, August 2017.

37. PwC, 'Women Returners: The £1 Billion Career Break Penalty for Professional Women', Online Insights Portal.

38. In the UK, a Mid-Life Career Review has been piloted by the National Institute of Adult Continuing Education. John Cridland recommended this should be offered to people in their late fifties or early sixties, but I think that is too late: see Cridland, John, 'Independent Review of the State Pension Age: Smoothing the Transition', HMG, Final Report, March 2017.

39. Barlow, John Perry, 'A declaration of the independence of cyberspace', Electronic Frontier Foundation.

40. Garnero, A., Kampelmann, S., Rycx, F., 'Part-time work, wages, and productivity: evidence from Belgian matched panel data', *ILR Review*, 2014, 67 (3), 926–54. Backes-Gellner, Uschi and Veen, Stephan, 'The impact of aging and age diversity on company performance', January 2009, https://ssrn.com/abstract=1346895. Ilmakunnas, P. and Ilmakunnas, S., 'Diversity at the workplace: whom does it benefit?', *De Economist*, 2011, 159, 223.

41. Börsch-Supan, Axel and Weiss, Matthias, 'Productivity and age: evidence from work teams at the assembly line', MEA Discussion Paper Series, 2011, no. 07148, Munich Center for the Economics of Aging (MEA) at the Max Planck Institute for Social Law and Social Policy.

42. CVS Caremark, 'Talent is Ageless', The Center on Aging and Work at Boston College.

43. Kunze, F., Boehm, S.A., Bruch, H., 'Age diversity, age discrimination climate and performance consequences – a cross organizational study', *Journal of Organizational Behavior*, 2011, 32, 264–90.

44. Lawrence, B.S, 'Age grading: the implicit organizational timetable', *Journal of Organizational Behavior*, 1984, 5, 23–35.

45. National Institute for Adult Continuing Education, 'Final report to the Department for Business, Innovation and Skills', July 2015.

46. Jossoff, Maya, 'Uber just released its first report on its drivers – here are the numbers', *Business Insider*, January 2015.

47. Auerbach, Alan J., et al., 'How the growing gap in life expectancy may affect retirement benefits and reforms', *The Geneva Papers on Risk and Insurance – Issues and Practice, The Geneva Association, 2017*, 42 (3), 475–99.

48. Milne, Richard, 'Finland's finance minister rejects universal basic income', *Financial Times*, 1 May 2018.

49. Couglan, Sean, 'Pisa tests: Singapore top in global education ranking', BBC News Online, 2018.

50. Singapore expects immigration to lead to a 20 per cent increase in population by 2050.

51. Cavendish, Camilla, 'The Cavendish Review', UK Department of Health, 2013.

52. Except at the Open University, an excellent institution which goes out of its way to teach mature students.

5. New Neurons

1. Tomas Bjork Eriksson found that terminal cancer patients in their fifties, sixties and seventies were still producing new neurons in their brains, and at an astonishing rate: between 500 and 1,000 neurons a day.

2. Nottebohm, F., 'A brain for all seasons', *Science*, Dec. 1981, 214, 1368–70.

3. In 1998 by Peter Eriksson and Frederick Gage.

4. Gage, F., 'Neurogenesis in the adult brain', *Journal of Neuroscience*, 2002, 22, 612–13.

5. Maguire, E.A., Woollett, K., Spiers, H.J., 'London taxi drivers and bus drivers: a structural MRI and neuropsychological analysis', *Hippocampus*, 2006, 16, 1091–101.

6. Kempermann, G., Kuhn, H.G., Gage, F.H., 'More hippocampal neurons in adult mice living in an enriched environment', *Nature, 1997, 386*, 493–5.

7. Van Praag, H., Christie, B.R., Sejnowski, T.J., Gage, F.H., 'Running enhances neurogenesis, learning and long term potentiation in mice', *Proceedings of the National Academy of Sciences USA*, 1999, 96 (23), 13427–31.

8. Colcombe, S.J., et al., 'Aerobic exercise training increases brain volume in aging humans', *Journals of Gerontology. Series A, Biological Sciences and Medical Sciences*, 2006, 61 (11), 1166–70.

9. Shors, T.J., et al., 'Use it or lose it: how neurogenesis keeps the brain fit for learning', *Behavioural Brain Research, 2011*, 227 (2), 450–58.

10. Van Praag, H., Kempermann, G, Gage, F.H., 'Running increases cell proliferation and neurogenesis in the adult mouse dentate gyrus', *Nature Neuroscience*, 1999, 2, 266–70.

11. Hanna-Pladdy, B., et al., 'The relation between instrumental musical activity and cognitive aging', *Neuropsychology*, 2011, 25, 378–86.

12. Merzenich, M.M., et al., 'Somatosensory cortical map changes following digit amputation in adult monkeys', *Journal of Comparative Neurology*, 1984, 224, 591–605.

13. UK Stroke Association, 'State of the Nation: Stroke Statistics', Report, February 2018.

14. Wolf, Steven L., Winstein, Carolee J., Miller, J. Philip, 'Effect of constraint-induced movement therapy on upper extremity function 3 to 9 months after stroke: the EXCITE randomized clinical trial', *Journal of the American Medical Association*, 2006, 296 (17), 2095–104.

15. The search for brain biomarkers is at an early stage, but might include the ability to preserve mutual inhibition between the two hemispheres of the brain, for example.

16. Doidge, Norman, *The Brain That Changes Itself* (New York: Penguin Books, 2007).

17. Wan, Catherine Y. and Schlaug, Gottfried, 'Music making as a tool for promoting brain plasticity across the life span', *The Neuroscientist*, 2010, 16 (5), 566-77.

18. Verghese J., Lipton R.B., Katz M.J., Hall C.B., Derby C.A., Kuslansky G., et al., 'Leisure activities and the risk of dementia in the elderly', *New England Journal of Medicine*, 2003, 348(25), 2508–16.

19. Gottlieb, S., 'Mental activity may help prevent dementia', *BMJ*, 2003, 326 (7404), 1418. Verghese, J., et al., 'Leisure activities and the risk of dementia in the elderly', *New England Journal of Medicine*, 2003, 348, 2508–16.

20. Staff, R.T., Hogan, M.J., Williams, D.S., Whalley, L.J., 'Intellectual engagement and cognitive ability in later life (the "use it or lose it" conjecture): longitudinal, prospective study', *BMJ*, 2018, 363, k4925. Pillai, J.A., Hall, C.B., et al., 'Association of crossword puzzle participation with memory decline in persons who develop dementia', *Journal of the International Neuropsychology Society*, 2011, 17 (6), 1006–13.

21. Snowdon, David, *Aging with Grace: The Nun Study and The Science of Old Age: How We Can All Live Longer, Healthier and More Vital Lives* (London: Fourth Estate, 2001).

22. SantaCruz, K.S., Sonnen, J.A., Pezhouh, M.K., Desrosiers, M.F., Nelson, P.T., Tyas, S.L., 'Alzheimer disease pathology in subjects without dementia in 2 studies of aging: the Nun Study and the 66 Adult Changes in Thought Study', *Journal of Neuropathology and Experimental Neurology*, 2011, 70, 832–40.

23. Riley, K.P., Snowdon, D.A., Desrosiers, M.F., Markesbery, W.R., 'Early life linguistic ability, late life cognitive function, and neuropathology: findings from the Nun Study', *Neurobiology of Aging*, 2005, 26 (3), 341–7.

24. Livingston, Gill, et al., 'Dementia prevention, intervention, and care', The Lancet Commission on Dementia, *Lancet*, 2017, 390 (10113).

25. Ibid.

26. Harvard Medical School, *A Guide to Cognitive Fitness*, Harvard Health Publishing, 2017.

27. US Federal Trade Commission, 'Lumosity to Pay $2 Million to Settle FTC Deceptive Advertising Charges for Its "Brain Training" Program', FTC Online, January 2016.

28. Stanford University Center on Longevity, 'A Consensus on the Brain Training Industry from the Scientific Community'.

29. Ibid.

30. Emamzedah, A., 'Evidence that computerized cognitive training works', *Psychology Today* Online, August 2018.

31. Simons, Daniel J., et al., 'Do brain training programs work?', *Psychological Science in the Public Interest*, October 2016.

32. Rebok, George W., et al., 'Ten-year effects of the advanced cognitive training for independent and vital elderly cognitive training trial on cognition and everyday functioning in older adults', *Journal of the American Geriatrics Society*, 2014, 62 (1), 16–24.

33. Simons, Daniel J., et al., 'Do "brain-training" programs work?', *Psychological Science in the Public Interest*, 2016, 17 (3), 103–86.

34. Yong, Ed., 'The weak evidence behind brain-training games', *The Atlantic*, 3 October 2016.

35. Edwards, Jerri D., et al., 'Speed of processing training results in lower risk of dementia', *Alzheimer's & Dementia (N.Y.)*, 2017, 3 (4), 603–11.

36. National Academies of Sciences, Engineering, and Medicine, *Preventing Cognitive Decline and Dementia: A Way Forward* (Washington, DC: The National Academies Press, 2017).

37. World Health Organization, Depression Factsheet.

38. Ma, S.H. and Teasdale, J.D., 'Mindfulness-based cognitive therapy for depression: replication and exploration of differential relapse prevention effects', *Journal of Consulting and Clinical Psychology*, 2004, 72, 31–40.

39. Goldapple, K., Segal, Z., et al., 'Modulation of cortical-limbic pathways in major depression: treatment-specific effects of cognitive behavior therapy', *Archives of General Psychiatry*, 2004, 61, 34–41.

40. Davidson, Richard J. and Lutz, Antoine, 'Buddha's brain: neuroplasticity and meditation', *IEEE Signal Processing Magazine*, 2008, 25 (1), 174–6.

41. Klingberg, Torkel, *The Overflowing Brain* (New York: Oxford University Press, 2009).

42. Harvard Medical School, 'More than sad: depression affects your ability to think', Blog Post.

43. Bullmore, Edward, *The Inflamed Mind* (London: Short Books, 2018).

44. Santarelli, L., et al., 'Requirement of hippocampal neurogenesis for the behavioral effects of antidepressants', *Science*, 2003, 301 (5634), 805–9.

45. 'Keyboard style could give early warning of dementia', *New Scientist*, 19 August 2009.

46. Klingberg, Torkel, *The Overflowing Brain* (New York: Oxford University Press, 2009).

47. Livingston, Gill, et al., 'Dementia prevention, intervention, and care', The Lancet Commission on Dementia, July 2017.

48. Alzhimer's Society, 'How to reduce your risk of dementia', Online Factsheet.

6. In the Genes

1. Okinawa Centenarian Study.

2. Mattison, Julie, et al., 'Caloric restriction improves health and survival of rhesus monkeys', *Nature Communications*, 2017, 8 (14063).

3. Wei, M., et al., 'Fasting-mimicking diet and markers/risk factors for aging, diabetes, cancer, and cardiovascular disease', *Science Translational Medicine*, 2017 9 (377), ii: eaai8700.

4. 'UNSW–Harvard scientists unveil a giant leap for anti-ageing', UNSW Sydney Newsroom, March 2017. Zhang, Hongbo, et al., 'NAD+ repletion improves mitochondrial and stem cell function and enhances life span in mice', *Science*, 2016, 352 (6292), 1436–43.

5. Dellinger, R. W., et al., 'Repeat dose NRPT (nicotinamide riboside and pterostilbene) increases NAD⁺ levels in humans safely and sustainably: a randomized, double-blind, placebo-controlled study', *Aging and Mechanisms of Disease*, 2017 3 (17).

6. 'Dietary supplements: Nobel or Ignoble', *Boston Globe*, 31 March 2017.

7. Kenyon, Cynthia, et al., 'A *C. elegans* mutant that lives twice as long as wild type', *Nature*, 1993, 366, 461–4.

8. Ohnishi, T., Mori, E., Takahashi, A., 'DNA double-strand breaks: their production, recognition, and repair in eukaryotes', *Mutation Research*, 2009, 669 (1–2), 8–12.

9. 'Jeanne Calment, world's elder, dies at 122', *New York Times*, 5 August 1997.

10. Watts, Geoff, 'Leonard Hayflick and the limits of ageing', *Lancet*, 2011, 377, 9783.

11. Bernardes de Jesus, B., Vera, E., Schneeberger, K., et al., 'Telomerase gene therapy in adult and old mice delays aging and increases longevity without increasing cancer', *EMBO Molecular Medicine*, 2012, 4 (8), 691–704.

12. Barbi, E., et al., 'The plateau of human mortality: demography of longevity pioneers', *Science*, 2018, 360, 1459–61.

13. Schoenhofen, Emily A., Wyszynski, Diego F., et al., 'Characteristics of 32 supercentenarians', *Journal of the American Geriatrics Society*, 2006, 54 (8), 1237–40.

14. 'Naked mole rats defy the biological law of aging', *Science*, 26 January 2018.

15. For a lengthier explanation see Mellon, Jim and Chalabi, Al, *Juvenescence: Investing in the Age of Longevity* (Douglas, IoM: Fruitful Publications, 2017).

16. Howitz, K.T., et al., 'Small molecule activators of sirtuins extend *Saccharomyces cerevisiae* lifespan', *Nature*, 2003, 425 (6954), 191–6.

17. 'Glaxo drops version of resveratrol "red wine" drug', Reuters, December 2010.

18. Bannister, C. A., Holden, S.E., et al., 'Can people with type-2 diabetes live longer than those without?', *Diabetes Obesity and Metabolism*, 2014, 16 (11), 1165–73.

19. TAME, 'Targeting Ageing With Metformin', Albert Einstein College of Medicine.

20. Silver, Dave, 'New Taiwan study contradicts earlier findings on Metformin's neurodegenerative disease protective effect', *Biotech East*, 31 March 2017.

21. Li, J, et al., 'A conserved NAD + binding pocket that regulates protein-protein interactions during aging', *Science*, 2017, 355 (6331), 1312–17.

22. Mannick, J.B., et al., 'mTOR inhibition improves immune function in the elderly', *Science Translational Medicine*, 2014, 6 (268), 268ra179.

23. Kennedy, Brian K. and Pennypacker, Juniper K., 'Ageing interventions get human', *Oncotarget Journal*, 2015, 6 (2), 590–91.

24. mTOR stands for 'Mechanistic target of rapamycin'.

25. 'Hope for thousands as stem-cell treatment restores eyesight', *The Times*, 20 March 2018.

26. Takahashi, K. and Yamanaka, S., 'Induction of pluripotent stem cells from mouse embryonic and adult fibroblast cultures by defined factors', *Cell*, 2006, 126 (4), 663–76.

27. Cookson, C., 'Experts warn on proliferation of dubious stem-cell clinics', *Financial Times*, 10 July 2018.

28. Olshansky, S.J., Carnes, B.A., Cassel, C., 'In search of Methuselah: estimating the upper limits to human longevity', *Science*, 1990, 250 (4981), 634–40.

29. Goldman, D.P., et al., 'Substantial health and economic returns from delayed aging may warrant a new focus for medical research', *Health Affairs*, 2013, 32 (10), 1698.

30. 'Here's what Bill Gates had to say in his latest Reddit "Ask Me Anything"', OnMSTF.com, 29 January 2015.

7. Out of the Ghetto

1. Rocco, L. and Suhrcke, M., *Is Social Capital Good for Health? A European Perspective* (Copenhagen: WHO Regional Office for Europe, 2012).

2. Holt-Lunstad et al, 'Social relationships and mortality risk: a meta-analytic review'. *PLoS Medicine,* 2010.

3. Holwerda, T.J., Deeg, D.J.H., et al., 'Feelings of loneliness, but not social isolation, predict dementia onset: results from the Amsterdam Study of the Elderly (AMSTEL)', *Journal of Neurology, Neurosurgery and Psychiatry,* 2014, 85 (2), 135–42.

4. Property Council of Australia–Retirement Living Council, 'National Overview of the Retirement Village Sector', October 2014.

5. Retirement Living Council Australia, 'Profile: Retirement Village Residents'.

6. Online Vimeo Video, 'Senior Cohousing: A Different Way of Living', https://vimeo.com/246241053.

7. Age UK, 'Later Life in the United Kingdom', April 2018.

8. English Housing Survey.

9. Age UK, 'Later Life in the United Kingdom', April 2018.

10. Cox, Hugo, 'The business of ageing: high-end housing for the elderly', *Financial Times* Online, January 2016.

11. National Union of Students, 'Almost half of 2015 graduates have moved back in with parents', Online Press Release.

12. 'A record 64 million Americans live in multigenerational houses', Pew Online, April 2018.

13. Ibid.

14. United Nations Department of Economic and Social Affairs, '68% of the world population projected to live in urban areas by 2050, says UN', Online News, May 2018.

15. 'Action Plans for Ageing Cities', Arup.com.

8. Health Revolution

1. 'The State of the Adult Social Care Sector and Workforce in England', Skills for Care, September 2018.

2. Cavendish, Camilla, 'The Cavendish Review', UK Department of Health, 2013.

3. Ibid.

4. maatschappelijke Business Case (mBC), Buurtzorg Nederland, 2009, Transitieprogramma.nl.

5. 'Shortage of nursing care workers', *Japan Times* Editorial, 7 July 2015.

6. 'Record 16,000 people with dementia went missing in 2017', *Japan Times*, 14 June 2018.

7. Carers Trust, 'Key Facts About Carers and the People They Care For', Online Factsheet.

8. Finkelstein, Amy and Brown, Jeffrey, 'Insuring long-term care in the United States', *Journal of Economic Perspectives*, 2011, 25 (4), 119–42.

9. 'As population ages, where are the geriatricians?', *New York Times*, 25 January 2016.

10. Fisher, J.M., Garside, M., Hunt, K., Lo, N., 'Geriatric medicine workforce planning: a giant geriatric problem or has the tide turned?', *Clinical Medicine*, 2014, 14 (2), 102–6.

11. Prince, M., et al., 'Dementia UK: Update', report produced by King's College London and the London School of Economics for the Alzheimer's Society, 2014.

9. Finding *Ikigai*

1. Age UK, 'Help us save free TV for older people!' Online Press Release, December 2018.

2. Gruenewald, Tara L., et al., 'Feelings of usefulness to others, disability, and mortality in older adults: The MacArthur Study of Successful Aging', *Journals of Gerontology: Series B, Psychological Sciences and Social Sciences*, 2007, 62 (1), 28–37.

3. Kim, Eric S., et al., 'Association between purpose in life and objective measures of physical function in older adults', *JAMA Psychiatry*, 2017, 74 (10), 1039–45.

4. Boyle, Patricia A., et al., 'Effect of a purpose in life on risk of incident Alzheimer disease and mild cognitive impairment in community-dwelling older persons', *Archives of General Psychiatry*, 2010, 67 (3), 304–10.

5. Chibanda, D., et al., 'Effect of a primary care-based psychological intervention on symptoms of common mental disorders in Zimbabwe: a randomized clinical trial', *Journal of the American Medical Association*, 2016, 316 (24), 2618–26.

6. www.friendshipbenchzimbabwe.org.

7. Fried, Linda, 'Making aging positive', *The Atlantic Online*, June 2014.

8. Rebok, G.W., Carlson, M.C., Glass, T.A., et al., 'Short-term impact of Experience Corps® participation on children and schools: results from a pilot randomized trial', *Journal of Urban Health*, 2004, 81 (1), 79–93.

9. Hong, S.I. and Morrow-Howell, Nancy, 'Health outcomes of Experience Corps®: a high-commitment volunteer program', *Social Science & Medicine*, 2010, 71 (2), 414–20.

10. Through the American Association for Retired Persons (AARP).

11. 'Study finds students with Experience Corps tutors make 60% more progress in critical reading skills than students without tutors', Washington University in St Louis, Online Article.

12. Not his real name.

13. UK Parliament, 'Social Insurance and Allied Services' (Beveridge Report).

14. Damian, R. I., et al., 'Sixteen going on sixty-six: a longitudinal study of personality stability and change across 50 years', *Journal of Personality and Social Psychology*, 2018, http://dx.doi.org/10.1037/pspp0000210.

10. Generation Hexed

1. I acknowledge that some pensioners still pay tax: my point is that overall, the balance has changed.

2. Pew Research Center, 'Angry Silents, Disengaged Millennials: The Generation Gap and the 2012 Election', November 2011.

3. Ipsos MORI, 5 September 2016.

4. Somerset Webb, Merryn, 'The Bank of Mum and Dad risks going out of business', *Financial Times*, 30 August 2018.

5. 'Passing On', *Resolution Foundation*, 2018, https://www.resolution foundation.org/app/uploads/2018/05/IC-inheritance-tax.pdf.

6. Resolution Foundation, 'A New Generational Contract', Resolution Foundation Intergenerational Commission Final Report, May 2018.

7. John C. Weicher, *The Distribution of Wealth in America, 1983–2013* (Hudson: 2017).

8. 'Recent Retirees Drive Pensioner Incomes Above Those of Working Families', Resolution Foundation, February 2017.

9. UK Office for National Statistics, 'PS: Net Debt (excluding public sector banks) as a % of GDP: NSA', Online Timeseries.

10. Lee, Ronald and Mason, Andrew, 'National transfer accounts', East-West Center.

11. Lee, Ronald and Mason, Andrew, *Population Aging and the Generational Economy: A Global Perspective* (Cheltenham: Edward Elgar, 2011).

12. 'Media starts to focus on Japan's aging prison population', *Japan Times*, 28 January 2017.

13. 'Crime in Japan', Custom Products Research Report.

14. Fukada, Shiho, 'Japan's prisons are a haven for elderly women', Bloomberg Online, March 2018.

15. Ibid.

16. Custom Products Research.

17. Age UK, 'Poverty In Later Life', Online Factsheet.

18. Dinkin, Elliot, '40% of the American middle class face poverty in retirement, study concludes', CNBC Online.

19. Collett, John, 'Grandparents stepping up as costs of childcare bite', *Sydney Morning Herald* Online, June 2018.

20. Glaser, K., Price, D., di Gessa, G., Ribe Montserrat, E., Tinker, A., *Grandparenting in Europe: Family Policy and Grandparents' Role in Providing Childcare* (Grandparents Plus, 2013).

21. '10 percent of grandparents live with a grandchild, Census Bureau reports', US Census Bureau, October 2014.

22. Shaw, Esther, 'No time for childcare grandparents to take it easy, they're worth £2,000 a year', *Guardian* Online, January 2016.

23. 'Retirement is out, new portfolio careers are in', *The Economist* Online, July 2017.

24. 'Older Americans provide services valued at $78 billion to U.S. economy', US Corporation for National and Community Service, 2017.

25. Gal, Robert I., Vanhuysse, Pieter, Vargha, Lili, 'Pro-elderly welfare states within child-oriented societies', *Journal of European Public Policy*, 2018, 25 (6), 944–58.

26. The Economist Intelligence Unit, 'Redrafting the Social Contract', *Swiss Life*, March 2016.

27. Emmerson, Carl, 'Would You Rather? Further Increases in the State Pension Age v Abandoning the Triple Lock', Institute for Fiscal Studies, 2017.

28. 'Passing On', *Resolution Foundation*, 2018.

Further Reading

Begley, Sharon. *The Plastic Mind: New Science Reveals Our Extraordinary Potential to Transform Ourselves*, Constable, 2009

Bullmore, Edward. *The Inflamed Mind: A Radical New Approach to Depression*, Short Books Limited, 2018

Cicero, Marcus Tullius. *How to Grow Old: Ancient Wisdom for the Second Half of Life*, Princeton University Press, 2016

Coughlin, Joseph P. *The Longevity Economy: Inside the World's Fastest-Growing, Most Misunderstood Market*, PublicAffairs, 2017

Doidge, Norman. *The Brain That Changes Itself: Stories of Personal Triumph from the Frontiers of Brain Science*, Penguin, 2008

Freedman, Marc. *Encore: Finding Work That Matters in the Second Half of Life*, PublicAffairs, 2008

Gawande, Atul. *Being Mortal: Illness, Medicine and What Matters in the End*, Wellcome Collection, Profile Books Limited, 2015

Goleman, Daniel. *Emotional Intelligence: Why It Can Matter More than IQ*, Bloomsbury, 1996

Gratton, Lynda and Scott, Andrew. *The 100-Year Life: Living and Working in an Age of Longevity*, Bloomsbury Business, 2017

Gray, Sir Muir. *Sod 70! The Guide to Living Well*, Bloomsbury Sport, 2015

Irving, Paul et al. *The Upside of Ageing: How Long Life Is Changing the World of Health*, John Wiley & Sons, 2014

James, Oliver. *Contented Dementia: A Revolutionary New Way of Treating Dementia: 24-Hour Wraparound Care for Lifelong Well-Being*, Vermilion, 2009

Jolivet, Muriel. *Japan: The Childless Society? The Crisis of Motherhood*, Routledge, 1997

Magnus, George. *The Age of Aging: How Demographics Are Changing the Global Economy and Our World*, John Wiley & Sons, 2008

Marmot, Michael. *The Health Gap: The Challenge of an Unequal World*, Bloomsbury Paperbacks, 2016

Mellon, Jim and Chalabi, Al. *Juvenescence: Investing in the Age of Longevity*, Fruitful Publications, 2017

Merzenich, Michael. *Soft-Wired: How the New Science of Brain Plasticity Can Change Your Life*, Parnassus Publishing, 2013

Snowdon, David. *Aging with Grace: The Nun Study and the Science of Old Age: How We Can All Live Longer, Healthier and More Vital Lives*, Fourth Estate, 2001

Taylor, Paul. *The Next America: Boomers, Millennials, and the Looming Generational Showdown*, PublicAffairs, 2016

Topol, Eric. *Topol Review: Preparing the Healthcare Workforce to Deliver the Digital Future*, Health Education England, 2019

Turkle, Sherry. *Alone Together: Why We Expect More from Technology and Less from Each Other*, Basic Books, 2017

Walker, Alan (ed.). *The New Science of Ageing*, Policy Press, 2014

Acknowledgements

I HAVE MET SO many wonderful, inspiring people in the course of writing this book who were generous with their time. They are too numerous to name, but I am especially grateful to the following for their support and insights: Jason Pontin at Flagship Pioneering; Paul Irving at the Milken Institute; Mark Henderson and Andrew Welchman at Wellcome Trust; Ambassadors Peter Wilson and Paul Madden; Rudiger van Leenan; Jan Kessler; Richard Lloyd Parry, Chie Matsumoto, Joshua Ogawa, Alec Russell, Eleanor Mills, Monique Charlesworth and my godfather, Bryan Magee, who at 88 has just published what he says is his last book – but hopefully will not be.

Particular thanks to Professors Jeff Liebman, John Haigh and Richard Zeckhauser at the Harvard Kennedy School and, most of all, Professor Larry Summers, without whom I would never have embarked on this.

Thanks also to Rohan Silva for giving me a second home, Emily Benn for tireless research assistance, Al Bowman and Robert Hands for shrewd comments on drafts, my wonderful agent Martin Redfern at Northbank, and my brilliant editor Ed Faulkner and the team at HarperCollins. And to Huw, Cosmo, Sasha and Ned, for putting up with my writing struggles, and my air miles, and for being the most wonderful family I could ever have.

The views and opinions expressed in this book, and any errors or oversights, are mine alone.

Index

Pager references in *italics* indicate images.